The Physician's Assistant—
Today and Tomorrow

The Physician's Assistant – Today and Tomorrow

Issues Confronting New Health Practitioners

Alfred M. Sadler, Jr.
Blair L. Sadler
Ann A. Bliss

Second Edition

Ballinger Publishing Company ● Cambridge, Mass.
A Subsidiary of J.B. Lippincott Company

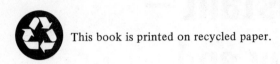

The first edition of this book was made possible in part by funds granted by:
the Carnegie Corporation, the Commonwealth Fund, the Foundation for Child
Development (formerly the Association for the Aid of Crippled Children), the
Josiah Macy Foundation, and the Rockefeller Foundation.

The statements made and views expressed are solely the responsibility of the
authors.

International Standard Book Number: 0–88410–125–8–Hbk.
0–88410–124–X–Pbk.

Library of Congress Catalog Card Number: 75–22407

Printed in the United States of America

Library of Congress Cataloging in Publication Data

Sadler, Alfred Mitchell, 1941–
   The physician's assistant—today and tomorrow.

   Bibliography: p.
   Includes index.
   1. Physicians' assistants—United States.
I. Sadler, Blair L., joint author. II. Bliss, Ann A.,
joint author. III. Title. [DNLM: 1. Physicians'
Assistants. W21.5 S126p]
R697.P45S23 1975   610.69'53   75–22407
ISBN 0–88410–125–8
ISBN 0–88410–124–X pbk.

Dedication

To Terrance Keenan and Margaret Mahoney who while at the Commonwealth Fund and the Carnegie Corporation nurtured the development of the new health practitioner concept.

Contents

List of Tables

List of Figures

Foreword

The authors, a physician, a lawyer, and a nurse, have combined their professional insights to provide a unique overview of issues confronting the newest health care professional—the physician's assistant. While recognizing the great promise of the PA for improved health care, they also highlight some of the many problems that lie ahead.

Aware of what the past can teach about the development of health professions, they raise issues of distribution, economics, education, task delegation, and protection of the public. Interdependent relationships of PA's with other health care professionals are advocated and the reorganization of health care workers into health teams is supported. The emerging PA profession is urged to circumvent prideful professionalism and to focus on improving patient care.

To anyone familiar with health care in America, it is clear that many issues facing the physician's assistant also plague the larger health care system. Although the authors do not profess to have simple "answers" to the numerous issues they raise, their candid analysis leads to carefully articulated recommendations. This timely and informative book should stimulate productive dialogue and investigation toward improved patient care.

> Kenneth M. Endicott, M.D.
> *Administrator*
> *Health Resources Administration*
> *Department of Health, Education*
> *and Welfare*

May 1, 1972

Authors' Note
to the Second Edition

Although there were many reasons to revise this book, the most obvious are that there are no copies left, the demand for it continues, and we believe that the analysis contained therein remains timely and important. Although there have been significant developments in this field during the past three years, the questions posed and the recommendations made in the first edition are still very much in the forefront today.

Many qualified applicants are unable to find a place in an American medical school. The Congress continues to struggle with some form of national health insurance. Our heavy reliance on foreign medical graduates is increasingly questioned. And nearly everyone is critical of our inability to provide more front-line primary care of reasonable quality to all Americans during a time of rapidly increasing costs. With the increasing production of family practice physicians, the appropriate training, utilization, and reimbursement of new health practitioners,[1] who can assist physicians to deliver primary care, is under heavy debate.

In addition to revising the text where appropriate, we have added a new chapter entitled, "Epilogue: New Health Practitioners in Evolution" (pp. 153–176). This chapter takes note of important events since 1972, discusses the lack of fit between the specialist physicians now produced and society's needs for generalists, and presents the new health practitioner as the human equivalent of a

---

1. In the Epilogue, we have adopted the terminology "new health practitioner" to encompass the health care providers described in this book. This represents the current solution to the search for the most appropriate label (see pp. 7–11). See Alfred M. Sadler, Jr., "The New Health Practitioner in Primary Care," *Journal of Medical Education* 49 (September 1974):845–848.

major new technology. A supplementary bibliography directs the reader to appropriate new source material. Resource documents and appendixes are included to support our analysis and to provide important reference information.

Having reviewed recent developments, and aware of the growing competition for funding, we believe it is important to restate our underlying thesis: *The introduction of a new practitioner into the health care system with the accompanying issues of identity, status, professionalism, authority, scope of practice, responsibility, degree of independence, and cost represents a major experiment in social change. As such, the experiment must continue to be funded for at least another decade if its impact on improved quality, access, and economies in delivering health care is to be determined.* What can be learned from the introduction of new health practitioners during the late 1960s and the 1970s should shed important light on how health care will be delivered in the 1980s and beyond.

A.M.S., Jr.
B.L.S.
A.A.B.

Princeton, New Jersey
May 1, 1975

Preface to the First Edition

The first edition of this book was an outgrowth of a "White Paper on the Physician's Assistant." The white paper was prepared at the request of five foundations[1] that have supported the development of new forms of health manpower to deliver quality medical care. Our charge was to take a fresh look at the place of the physician's assistant[2] in American medicine, discuss the implications of this emerging new health professional, and identify important issues of value in directing further foundation research.

Following a meeting with the participating foundations in April 1971, during which our charge was defined, the study was accomplished through literature review, telephone discussions, meetings with individuals in the health manpower field, and our own analysis of available information and experience. Preliminary drafts of the paper were reviewed at meetings with foundation representatives in October and November 1971. A final draft was submitted on January 15, 1972.

Subsequently the paper was revised and expanded for publication as a book. The recommendations refer to what we believe is needed in the health manpower field generally. They reflect our views and are not necessarily the views of the foundations.

Of necessity, the first edition was prepared in the interstices of major commitments to the authors' principal activity at that

1. The Carnegie Corporation, the Commonwealth Fund, the Foundation for Child Development, the Josiah Macy Foundation, and the Rockefeller Foundation.
2. As in the first edition, the term "physician's assistant" includes a range of midlevel health workers variously named—physician's associates (Duke and related models), medex, nurse clinicians, nurse practitioners, physician extenders, child health associates, etc. Since the first edition, the term "new health practitioner" has become widely accepted as the generic term.

time, the Trauma Program of the Yale University School of Medicine. Given the constraints of time and our own work commitments, we did not attempt to provide detailed solutions to the issues, but endeavored to raise the right questions and to suggest productive approaches to their resolution.

Any attempt to fashion a rational view of health manpower risks reducing complex issues to simplistic generalizations. We may appear to be unreasonably critical of the positions of others, achieved often after long and hard work. We do not mean to imply that the assumptions under scrutiny are invalid; our aim, rather, is to delineate other lines of reasoning and points of view that should also be explored. We attempt to show, for example, that assumptions which were appropriate for one time and place simply do not obtain today.

We begin by reviewing briefly the physician's assistant phenomenon, its great promise to American health care, and the ample manpower resources for its growth and development ("Introduction"). Next ("Some Fundamental Concerns"), we address issues of timely import to the success of the PA:

1. levels, ratings, and titles,
2. co-option into specialty practice settings,
3. dependence vs. independence,
4. equality for the sexes,
5. methods of reimbursement.

The nursing profession is examined because of its relevance to the physician's assistant ("Lessons from Nursing"). We then move to issues which are likely to be framed in legal terms or resolved through the legal process ("Where the Law Intervenes"). Further, we explore briefly a variety of organizational settings which will affect the physician's assistant ("Organizational Alternatives") and we provide recommendations for action ("Issues and Recommendations"). A "Selected Bibliography" follows and material of special relevance is included in the "Appendixes."

ACKNOWLEDGMENTS

In preparing the first edition, we received generous assistance and advice from numerous individuals involved in health care and health manpower. The following people provided helpful insights and information: Martin Eggleston and Dr. Robert Farrier (American Hospital Association); Betty Jane Anderson, Joyce Burger, Donald

Foy, Naomi Patchin, and Dr. William Ruhe (American Medical Association); Pearl Dunkely (American Nurses Association); Dr. John A. D. Cooper, Joseph Keyes, and Dr. August Swanson (Association of American Medical Colleges); Dr. Henry Silver (University of Colorado Medical School); Eleanor Lambertsen (Cornell University School of Nursing); Dr. Louis Pondy (Duke University School of Business Administration); Dr. Eugene A. Stead (Duke University School of Medicine); Dr. Alfred Yankauer (Harvard School of Public Health); Dr. John Proffitt (HEW Office of Education); Mary Mac-Donald (Massachusetts General Hospital); Dr. John Hogness (National Academy of Sciences, Institute of Medicine); Madelyn Ferrigan and Dr. Edithe Levit (National Board of Medical Examiners); Rita Chow (National Center for Health Services Research and Development, HSMHA); Dr. Jerome Lysaught and Dr. Charles Russell (National Commission for the Study of Nursing and Nursing Education); Dr. Frank Dickey (National Commission on Accrediting); Mary Dineen (National League for Nursing); Dr. Nicholas Danforth and Dr. Bella Strauss (New England Medex Program); Veronica Driscoll and Cathryne Welsh (New York State Nurses Association); Dr. Warren Perry (State University of New York at Buffalo); Ellen Fahy (State University of New York at Stony Brook, School of Nursing); Dr. Kenneth Endicott, Gretchen Osgood, and Maryland Pennell (NIH, Bureau of Health Manpower Education); Dr. Lester Lave (Carnegie-Mellon University Graduate School of Industrial Administration); Karen Grimm, Dr. Jerry Miller, and Dr. William Selden (SASHEP); Dr. Mark Musser and Martha Phillips (Veterans Administration); Dr. Richard A. Smith (University of Washington Medical School); Margaret Arnstein, Laverne Fakkema, and Virginia Henderson (Yale University School of Nursing); Dr. Jack Cole, Paul Moson, and Dr. Alvin Novack (Yale University School of Medicine). Patricia Pac, a third year law student at Suffolk University, provided helpful and important research. Judy Castellon, Mary Beth Graham, and Linda Parkes provided invaluable aid in typing the numerous drafts of the manuscript.

We benefitted immeasurably from reviewing our ideas with representatives from the five foundations that supported our work. They included: Nora Piore and Dr. Robert Slater (Foundation for Child Development); Margaret Mahoney and Carol Richards (Carnegie Corporation); Dr. Reginald Fitz, Dr. Robert Glaser, Terrance Keenan, and Quigg Newton (The Commonwealth Fund); Dr. Vernon Lippard (Macy Foundation); and Dr. Guy Hayes, Thelma Ingles, and Dr. Willoughby Lathem (Rockefeller Foundation). We are particularly grateful to Miss Ingles, Mr. Keenan, Dr. Lippard, Miss Mahoney,

and Dr. Slater for their detailed editorial and conceptual assistance.
We extend special appreciation to Dr. Douglas A. Fenderson and Thomas Hatch (NIH, Bureau of Health Manpower Education) and Dr. Edmund Pellegrino (State University of New York School of Medicine, Stony Brook) for the generous sharing of their thoughts, recommendations, and insights, as well as their review of the draft manuscript. Without their help and support, this book would not have been possible. However, final and full responsibility for all statements and recommendations herein are ours alone.

A.M.S., Jr.
B.L.S.
A.A.B.

New Haven, Connecticut
May 1, 1972

The Physician's Assistant—
Today and Tomorrow

Chapter One

Introduction

THE PHYSICIAN'S ASSISTANT PHENOMENON

In many respects, the birth and development of the "physician's assistant" is the most exciting health manpower innovation in several decades.[1] It has highlighted the established belief that many tasks performed only by physicians can be carried out with equal competence by specially trained health professionals.

The PA concept is exciting because it holds great promise for improving and distributing health care. Many of the problems and issues which at first appear unique to the PA are, in fact, part of the most crucial issues affecting our health care system. Its development emphasizes the importance of these issues and helps to generate fresh insights into traditional and often moribund analyses.[2]

Although in 1971 less than 200 physician's assistants had been graduated, the public and professional interest in them was phenomenal.[3] The Department of Health, Education and Welfare

---

1. The American Medical Association's Board of Trustees and its Council on Health Manpower have recommended the following working definition of the "physician's assistant": "The physician's assistant is a skilled person qualified by academic and practical training to provide patient service under the supervision and direction of a licensed physician who is responsible for the performance of that assistant."
2. We will not use a personal pronoun when discussing the physician's assistant. Except for certain programs like Medex, which originally limited entry to the military corpsman, the masculine or feminine is equally appropriate.
3. Department of Health Manpower, Division of Medical Practice, American Medical Association, *1971 Survey of Operational "Physician's Assistant" Programs: Numbers Graduated and Employed* (August 1971). This figure does not include the graduates of nurse-expansion programs.

reported that 80 PA training programs were in various stages of development in addition to approximately 50 programs that extended nursing roles.[4]

A major federal commitment to train physician's assistants has been made. In his Health Message of February 18, 1971, President Nixon called for $15 million for the training of physician's assistants.[5] Following the president's lead, Congress passed the Comprehensive Health Manpower Training Act of 1971 which included explicit provision for the training of physician's assistants. In addition, funds authorized by the Health Training Improvement Act of 1970 and the Nurse Training Act of 1971 were earmarked for this purpose. To assure a unified approach, funding for physician's assistant programs was combined in the Office of Special Programs, Bureau of Health Manpower Education, National Institutes of Health, (see pp. 21–24).

The three branches of the armed services have developed physician's assistant programs.[6] The Veterans Administration has made a major training commitment,[7] and the Civil Service Commission has developed rating standards for various "levels" of physician's assistants.[8]

The public media have also shown considerable interest.

4. U.S. Department of Health, Education and Welfare, National Institutes of Health, *Selected Training Programs for Physician Support Personnel* (1971).

5. The President stated: "One of the most promising ways to expand the supply of medical care and to reduce its costs is through a greater use of allied health personnel, especially those who work as physician's and dentist's assistants, nurse pediatric practitioners and nurse midwives. Such persons are trained to perform tasks which must otherwise be performed by doctors themselves, even though they do not require the skills of a doctor. Such assistance frees a physician to focus his skills where they are most needed and often allows him to treat many additional patients." The President's Health Message (1971), p. 9.

6. *Air Force:* The first class of 25 students began on July 1, 1971. Located at Shephard Air Force Base, Wichita Falls, Texas, the 24 month course includes 12 months of academic study and 12 months preceptorship.
Army: The first class of 60 students began in February 1972. Located at Fort Sam Houston and affiliated with Baylor University, the course resembles the Air Force program in length and general structure.
Navy: The first class started in the summer of 1972. The program has been affiliated with the George Washington University School of Medicine.

7. The Veterans Administration has detailed a "routine work assignment" for utilizing the physician's assistant in the hospital setting in the VA Circular 10–71–32 entitled "Physician's Assistants—Guidelines for Utilization."

8. The Civil Service grades vary from GS–7 through GS–11, depending on background and education. United States Civil Service Commission, *Bridging the Medical Care Gap*, Announcement no. 428, March 1971.

The weekly magazines (*Time, Life,* etc.), a cartoon ("Gasoline Alley"), and television ("The Bold Ones", "Marcus Welby, M.D.," "Medical Center") have all featured the physician's assistant. The PA has been a political bonanza. Legislators have introduced a variety of "physician's assistant laws" in more than 40 states (see pp. 93–99 and Appendix B). The political appeal of providing a useful civilian health occupation for the returning Viet Nam medical corpsman was enormous. After initial reticence, the AMA joined in support of the PA and issued full page advertisements in national newspapers and magazines. Numerous meetings and conferences have discussed the arrival of the PA on the health scene.

THE PROMISE

Considering that a mere 200 physician's assistants existed in 1971, what explained the success of the PA in capturing the imagination of health professionals and the public? What place will the physician's assistant find in our already crowded constellation of manpower categories? *Answers to these questions reside in the following major promises—promises that may not necessarily be realized:*
    1. The physician's assistant is viewed as a creative solution to our health manpower shortage. The doctor deficit is one of the most discussed and documented aspects of our current health scene. Numerous efforts are under way to shorten the medical curriculum, develop varied and more flexible "track systems," expand medical school size, and create new schools. Indeed, the Carnegie Commission report outlined a massive plan to educate 50 percent more physicians by 1980.[9]
    For any of these efforts to be successful, the effectiveness of practicing physicians must also be maximized. Studies have demonstrated that much of what a physician does during his evaluation and care for patients is routine and repetitious and can be assumed by specially trained personnel. A detailed patient history, a physical examination, and many diagnostic and therapeutic procedures can all be performed competently, and in some cases more effectively, by well-trained persons who have time to devote to them.[10]

    9. Carnegie Commission on Higher Education, *Higher Education and the Nation's Health: Policies for Medical and Dental Education* (New York: McGraw–Hill, 1970).
    10. For example, see Charles E. Lewis, Barbara A. Resnik, Glenda Schmidt, and David Waxman, "Activities, Events and Outcomes in Ambulatory Patient Care," *New England Journal of Medicine* 280, no. 12 (March 20, 1969):645–49; Alfred Yankauer, John P. Connelly, and Jacob J. Feldman,

2. At a time when we were fighting an unpopular war, physician's assistant programs promised civilian jobs to experienced returning military servicemen. The designers of the physician's assistant concept recognized that a large manpower pool was available from the military services. Approximately 30,000 men who had some medical experience were being discharged each year. Of those, 6,000 had extensive medical training and independent duty experience.[11] Such individuals typically had been lost to our credential-happy civilian health care system because of their lack of formal education. Physician's assistant programs promised to help translate these hard-earned skills into useful civilian functions.

3. The soaring costs of medical education can be checked and even reduced by the use of a physician's assistant who can be trained in a relatively short period of time. Clearly it is much less expensive to train a physician's assistant over a two year span than to train one physician over an eight to ten year period. Although some medical schools now give the MD degree after three years, an additional three to six years are required for the training of a physician specialist.

4. Physician services which can be provided by nonphysicians should save the consumer money. As alternative payment schemes, such as prepaid group practice, are devised, the cost of medical care can be reduced through the utilization of less costly personnel.

5. The physician's assistant can contribute to quality medical care by allowing more patients to be seen under more optimal conditions. Less hurried examinations should provide more accurate diagnoses and permit the physician to concentrate on those patients who require his special knowledge and skills. The PA can also help to increase quality of care by freeing physician time to participate in continuing education and study.[12] Some physicians may not utilize such free time for continuing education and would prefer instead to relax and enjoy whatever extra moments are made available. If this leads to greater physician longevity, we will have

"Physician Productivity in the Delivery of Ambulatory Care," *Medical Care* 8 no. 1 (January–February 1970):35–46; K. D. Rogers, M. Mally, and F. L. Marcus, "A General Medical Practice Using Nonphysician Personnel," *Journal of the American Medical Association* 206, no. 8 (November 18, 1968):1753–57; Louis R. Pondy, "Physician's Assistant Productivity: Ayden, North Carolina" (Unpublished, Duke University, Durham, North Carolina, April 1970).

11. Richard A. Smith, "Medex—A Demonstration Program in Primary Medical Care," *Northwest Medicine* 68 (1969):1023–30.

12. Eugene A. Stead, "The Duke Plan for Physician's Assistants," *Medical Times* 95, no. 1 (January 1967):40–48.

helped to preserve the highest level of medical manpower resource.

6. The physician's assistant is viewed as providing more manpower for primary, preventive, and emergency care needs. With our increasing emphasis on specialization and subspecialization, most physicians are being educated beyond primary and general practice functions. The development toward subspecialization is understandable because with advancing technology, the explosion of medical knowledge, and the expansion of highly sophisticated medical centers, better care can be provided for complex medical problems. But in our rush to specialization, primary, preventive, and emergency care have been neglected.

PA MANPOWER SOURCES: A POOL OR AN OCEAN?

The physician's assistant movement has another important point in its favor. In addition to the previously cited Viet Nam veteran manpower pool, large reservoirs of highly intelligent, motivated individuals, with extensive health care experience, see being a PA as an attractive entrée to direct patient care. For many, direct patient care is where the action is in the health field. The PA concept provides the opportunity for students to get into patient care without the long, arduous, and expensive training commitment that is required of a physician.

The potential number of physician's assistants from the following variety of sources is substantial:

1. In 1970 alone, 24,987 people applied to U.S. medical schools with space for only 11,348.[13] According to the Association of American Medical Colleges, as many as one-half of the remaining 13,639 were "fully qualified" to become physicians. Many might be eager and able to deliver excellent primary health care as a PA if given the opportunity.

2. Other college graduates with outstanding records are not interested in lengthy training toward a medical subspecialty career and never even apply to medical school. Many would like to earn a living while serving their fellow man, and find in the PA an ideal career.

3. Some of the 700,000 employed registered nurses (500,000 full time and 200,000 part time) are excited about the possibility of both expanding their role and increasing job satisfac-

---

13. W. F. Dube, Frank T. Stritter, and Bonnie C. Nelson, "Study of U.S. Medical School Applicants, 1970–71," *Journal of Medical Education* 46, no. 10 (October 1971), p. 837.

tion by becoming physician's assistants. This may be their only way to overcome the rigid barriers to expanded function and increased financial reward.

4. Some of the more than 650,000 registered nurses "in retirement" might be induced back to work by programs offering increased opportunity and responsibility in primary patient care.[14]

5. Other health care professionals (e.g., pharmacists, inhalation therapists, laboratory technologists) see the PA as a way out of dead-end career patterns and into more active patient care management.

Thus, when considering the potentials and problems of the PA on the American health care scene, it would be myopic to focus discussion only on the returning military veteran or any other single group. Indeed, the military source has become less significant than the others outlined above. Applications to PA programs confirm the wide diversity of manpower sources.[15]

In summary, PAs, although originally few in number, are now being produced in quantity. We must continue to plan for the full impact of their arrival on the health scene.

---

14. In a survey of 90 baccalaureate graduate nurses from the University of Virginia, 88 percent approved of the primary care role for nurses, 65 percent desired such a role for themselves, 51 percent believed primary care would reactivate the nonpracticing nurse, and 70 percent would enroll in a primary care training program of up to nine months duration. Regina McCormack and Ronald Crawford, "Attitudes of Professional Nurses Toward Primary Care," *Nursing Research* 18 no. 6 (November–December 1969):542–44.

15. For example, requests for applications to the Yale Physician's Associate Program are being received at the rate of 50 per week.

Chapter Two

Some Fundamental Concerns

A ROSE BY ANY OTHER NAME

The development of a wide variety of PA programs throughout the nation has spawned a bewildering array of titles covering a broad spectrum of programs ranging from four months to five years. The following examples demonstrate the diversity.

1. Established in 1965, the Duke Physician's Assistant Program (now Physician's Associate) was originally designed to train assistants to overworked general practitioners.[1] The 24 month program, developed by Dr. Eugene Stead, Professor of Medicine, now offers its graduates a range of options in primary and specialty care.[2]

2. The University of Washington's Medex program was founded in 1969 for the returning military corpsman with extensive medical training and independent duty experience. Developed by Dr. Richard Smith, Associate Professor of Preventive Medicine, the program includes three months of university-based education followed by twelve months of preceptorship with a practicing physician. The objective is to mold each Medex to a particular physician's practice. Emphasis is placed on primary care practice in rural areas.[3]

3. The orthopedic assistant (1969) and urologic physician's assistant (1970) are examples of two year programs designed

---

1. Eugene A. Stead, "Conserving Costly Talents—Providing Physicians New Assistants," *Journal of the American Medical Association* 198, no. 10 (December 5 1966):1108–09.

2. E. Harvey Estes and D. Robert Howard, "Potential for New Classes of Personnel: Experiences of the Duke Physician's Assistant Program," *Journal of Medical Education* 45, no. 3 (March 1970):149–55.

3. Richard A. Smith, "MEDEX," *Journal of the American Medical Association* 211, no. 16 (March 16, 1970):1843–45.

to train personnel to work directly for specialists. These pilot programs, located in San Francisco and Cincinnati, respectively, were received with enthusiasm by the medical specialty societies concerned.

4. A four month "health assistants" training program is sponsored by Project Hope in Laredo, Texas (1970). The only requirement for entry is that the student be eighteen years of age. (Many students who lack high school diplomas also earn their General Equivalency Diploma Certificate upon completion of the program.)

5. The Pediatric Nurse Practitioner Program, inaugurated at the University of Colorado in 1965 by Dr. Henry Silver, Professor of Pediatrics, offers supervised opportunities for baccalaureate nurses to assume much of well-baby care and the management of simple pediatric illnesses, previously performed only by pediatricians. Four months of training are required.[4]

6. The Child Health Associate Program (1969), also developed by Dr. Silver, prepares individuals to "practice pediatrics" under close physician supervision as defined under a new Colorado law. Students are admitted after two years of college for a three year sequence of professional studies, including a year of internship. A baccalaureate degree is awarded.[5]

7. A variety of postbaccalaureate (certificate and master's) nurse practitioner programs are designed to expand nursing practice and encompass areas traditionally reserved only for the physician. Although these nurse-expansion programs are not officially designated "physician's assistant," they represent somewhat analogous attempts to expand the functions of experienced health personnel in direct patient care areas. Nurse practitioners are trained in one to two years to acquire "physician-like" skills and work under physician supervision.[6]

Efforts Toward a Consensus

In 1970 the National Congress on Health Manpower (sponsored by the AMA's Council on Health Manpower) sought to develop uniform terminology for the many emerging PA programs.

---

4. Henry K. Silver, Loretta C. Ford, and S. C. Stearly, "Program to Increase Health Care for Children: Pediatric Nurse Practitioner Program," *Pediatrics* 39, no. 5 (May 1967):756–60.

5. Henry K. Silver and James A. Hecker, "The Pediatric Nurse Practitioner and the Child Health Associate: New Types of Health Professionals," *Journal of Medical Education* 45, no. 3 (March 1970):171–76.

6. See Appendix A for the most recent list of physician's assistant and nurse practitioner programs.

The Congress concluded that "physician's assistant" was too general to be adopted as the single generic term because PAs were receiving varied levels of training. They decided that "associate" would be more appropriate for those health workers who assume a direct and responsible role in patient care and act as colleagues to physicians, rather than as their technical assistants. The Congress also noted that the physician's assistant terminology was often confused with the established "medical assistant," the title for the nonprofessional office helper who functions in a clerical and technical fashion.[7] In contrast, the AMA's House of Delegates rejected the "associate" terminology in the belief that "associate" should be applied only to physicians working in collaboration with other physicians. (This criticism ignored the apostrophe "s" which denotes that the "associate" is not another physician.) Thus, no consistent position has emerged from organized medicine.

In 1970 the Board on Medicine of the National Academy of Sciences classified physician's assistants according to the degree of specialization and level of judgment. The Board's report stated:

> The Type A assistant is capable of approaching the patient, collecting historical and physical data, organizing the data, and presenting them in such a way that the physician can visualize the medical problem and determine appropriate diagnostic or therapeutic steps. He is also capable of assisting the physician by performing diagnostic and therapeutic procedures and coordinating the roles of other more technical assistants. While he functions under the general supervision and responsibility of the physician, he might under special circumstances and under defined rules, perform without the immediate surveillance of the physician. He is, thus distinguished by his ability to integrate and interpret findings on the basis of general medical knowledge to exercise a degree of independent judgment.
>
> The Type B assistant, while not equipped with general knowledge and skills relative to the whole range of medical care, possesses exceptional skill in one clinical specialty or, more commonly, in certain procedures within such a specialty. In his area of specialty, he has a degree of skill beyond that normally possessed by a Type A assistant and perhaps that normally possessed by physicians who are not engaged in the specialty. Because his knowledge and skill are limited to a particular specialty, he is less qualified for independent action. An example of this type of assistant might be one who is highly skilled in the physician's functions associated with a renal

---

7. For example, the terms "medical assistant" and "physician's assistant" appear to be used interchangeably in an article by William J. Curran, "Legal Responsibility for Actions of Physician's Assistants," *New England Journal of Medicine* 286, no. 5 (February 1972):254.

dialysis unit and who is capable of performing these functions as required.

The Type C assistant is capable of performing a variety of tasks over the whole range of medical care under the supervision of a physician, although he does not possess the level of medical knowledge necessary to integrate and interpret findings. He is similar to a Type A assistant in the number of areas in which he can perform, but he cannot exercise the degree of independent synthesis and judgment of which Type A is capable. This type of assistant would be to medicine what the practical nurse is to nursing.

The NAS classification was helpful but also caused some confusion. Dr. Harvey Estes of Duke, writing in *Modern Medicine*, assigned a Type A rating to the Duke graduate and labeled the Medex a Type C.[8] This aroused considerable consternation among Medex leaders who believe that their graduates are trained to an equal level of performance, although by a different process. In drafting essentials for the "Assistant to the Primary Care Physician," the AMA rated the Duke PA and the Medex equally (see pp. 25–33).

Several PA programs training individuals to work as colleagues of physicians have chosen the name physician's associate. Such programs (e.g., Yale and Duke) believe that "associate" more effectively describes a functioning health team and indicates a more collaborative relationship than the term assistant. Dorothy Mereness, Dean, University of Pennsylvania School of Nursing, agreed and said: "When two professional colleagues are functioning together as associates, they collaborate on decision-making and each has some responsibility for formulating the decision. When one person has the title of assistant in relation to a second individual, he carries out the decisions of the other." Physician's associates, of course, still function under the supervision and control of the physician and are responsible to him.[9]

The American Academy of Pediatrics proposed three titles representing a graded increase in competence and responsibility. They were pediatric aide, pediatric office assistant, and pediatric nurse associate.[10] Dr. Henry Silver suggested a new term for health personnel who perform physician-like tasks: "syniatrist" from the Greek "syn" signifying "along with" or "association" and "-iatric"

8. E. Harvey Estes, Jr., "The Training of Physician's Assistants: A New Challenge for Medical Education," *Modern Medicine* 38 (June 29, 1970): 90–93.

9. Dorothy Mereness, "Recent Trends in Expanding Roles of the Nurse," *Nursing Outlook* 18, no. 5 (May 1970):30–33.

10. American Academy of Pediatrics, Allied Health Workers in Pediatric Practice (September 1969), Evanston, Illinois.

which means "relating to medicine" or a "physician."[11] He modified the syniatrist terminology by a prefix relating to each medical specialty; for example, general practice, pediatrics, orthopedics. He specified the level to which the syniatrist is trained by using aide, assistant, and associate as suffixes. Thus, one could be an orthopedic syniatrist associate or a general practice syniatrist aide, etc. The term syniatrist would not be applied to such health professionals as laboratory technicians, medical office assistants, and X-ray technicians who do not perform physicianlike tasks or do not provide direct health care to patients.

The World Health Organization believes that such terms as assistant, auxiliary, or aide are demeaning and should be avoided.[12] Dr. Richard Smith of Seattle agrees. He created a new name (Medex) for his program and, in a *JAMA* article, presented a cluster of companion titles such as Osler, Flexner, and Cruzer.[13] He believes all are neutral and are not inherently demeaning.

In summary, the levels of training and competence and the associated names are confusing. But, it is not yet wise to insist upon a hierarchy of levels and a uniform nomenclature until more is understood about the consequences of such choices to health care. To settle upon a hierarchy of levels might result in premature closure in a field that clearly needs more research and evaluation.

THE PHYSICIAN'S ASSISTANT—
A TWENTIETH CENTURY JONAH?

Immediately upon graduation, the physician's assistant is in considerable danger of being swallowed whole by the whale that is our present entrepreneurial, subspecialty medical practice system. The likely co-option of the newly minted physician's assistant by subspecialty medicine is one of the most serious issues confronting the PA.

Although the greatest needs for improved care are in the areas of primary, preventive, and emergency medicine, a PA graduate will be tempted to move into specialty areas. The temptation is largely financial. PAs can start at $15,000 per year if they join a

11. Henry K. Silver, "The Syniatrist," *Journal of the American Medical Association* 217, no. 10 (September 6, 1971):1368–70.

12. World Health Organization, Technical Report Series 212 (1961), p. 26.

13. Richard A. Smith, Gerald R. Bassett, Carnick A. Markarian, Raymond E. Vath, William L. Freeman and G. Fredrick Dunn, "A Strategy for Health Manpower: Reflections on an Experience Called MEDEX," *Journal of the American Medical Association* 217, no. 10 (September 6, 1971):1362–67.

specialist's practice. In contrast, employment in an institutional setting—e.g., the emergency department outpatient clinic or neighborhood health clinic, may offer a lower salary. If nurses enter hospital work at $8,000 to $10,000, it is unlikely that PAs will receive much more in that setting. Health maintenance organizations and new primary care centers may offer more but can they afford to compete with private practice?

The Medex program in Seattle seeks to prevent co-option in two ways. First, preference is given to applicants from rural backgrounds who express a desire to return there. Second, following a year's preceptorship with an individual physician who is providing primary care in rural settings, the Medex is expected to be hired by the preceptor. Because the training physicians are specially selected general practitioners, there is an excellent opportunity for the Medex to remain in primary care and in geographical areas of shortage.

The graduates of the Duke Physician's Associate Program have no such direct tie to primary care and general practice, although the program has been billed as training individuals for these areas. Thus, until large numbers of physician's assistants are produced, the first to emerge will be in such demand that relatively few may end up in primary care or rural settings where the need is the greatest. The same may be said for inner city or poverty areas. The problem is compounded by the fact that the PA's professional role is directly linked to physicians, who are not only poorly distributed but have paid little attention to primary and emergency care. Few neighborhood health centers or clinics will be able to match the high salaries of the specialist's private office.

Although the deployment system of the Medex program helps prevent the co-option of each Medex by subspecialty practice, there are some disadvantages. Because the majority of Medex training is provided by one physician in one practice setting, the occupational mobility of each Medex may be limited. If the "preceptor physician" dies or retires, the Medex may not be readily employable in other settings without an additional preceptorship or training.[14] Because solo physician practice is yielding to prepaid health clinics and health maintenance organizations, training for PAs should include exposure to health care teams that can function in new organizations (see Chapter Five, "Organizational Alternatives").

Consequently, we believe that the distribution and placement of physician's assistants in primary and emergency care needs

---

14. Dr. Richard Smith disagrees. He believes that practicing primary care physicians are more likely to hire a Medex trained by another practicing physician than a Medex trained in an academic medical center environment (personal communication).

analysis and support. One solution might be to provide financial incentives for physician's assistants to work in areas of acute shortage in primary care. There are precedents for financial incentives in the federal legislation which has provided loan forgiveness and special scholarships to physicians who work in areas of great need. The Division of Nursing of the Bureau of Health Manpower of the Health Resources Administration has done the same. Such plans contain only a moral obligation to pay back loans. There is no way to enforce the location of practice. Administrators of these programs have been skeptical of the impact of loan forgiveness because of the strong pressures to work in areas of high economic reward.

As an alternative, some form of special stipend or income assurance mechanisms could be developed. An income assurance plan could underwrite the differential between what physician's assistants earn in a rural or shortage area of primary care and what they might earn in a comparable specialty setting. These are merely examples, and all possible remunerative mechanisms should be explored.

The use of multimedia communication links between geographically remote practice settings and university medical centers may equal financial inducements for encouraging rural practice. Further, the problem-oriented medical record[15] for self-assessment provides an important reinforcement for individuals working in isolated areas, far removed from peer review and the advantages of daily interchange with colleagues.

The National Health Service Corps was established under the Emergency Health Personnel Act of 1970 (PL 91–623) to alleviate the maldistribution of health services. By February 1972, 28 physicians, 10 dentists, 18 nurses and 12 supporting health professionals had been assigned to 18 communities designated as critical health manpower shortage areas by the Health Services and Mental Health Administration.[16] Additional personnel and shortage areas have been designated.

Recruitment for the National Health Service Corps has been difficult. According to the Corps' recruitment office, the major incentive for doctors to join has been fulfillment of military obligation. All 28 physicians in the first group were recruited from the U.S.

---

15. Lawrence L. Weed, "Medical Records that Guide and Teach," *New England Journal of Medicine* 278, no. 11 (March 14, 1968):593–600.
16. The original 18 designated areas were: Tuskegee, Alabama; Livingston and Sacramento (Isleton), California; Immokalee and Belle Glade, Florida; Chicago, Illinois; Leslie County, Kentucky; New Orleans, Louisiana; Jackman, Maine; Cato, Rochester and two sections of South Bronx, New York; Snow Shoe, Pennsylvania; Federal Way, Washington (Small Tribes Organization of Western Washington, Inc.); Glenville, West Virginia; and Menominee County, Wisconsin.

Public Health Service and many were still satisfying military requirements. An additional recruiting challenge has been to provide the
proper mix of personnel required by varied local needs. Appropriately, some health team members have been recruited at the local
level. The act authorized $20 million for fiscal 1972 and $30 million
for fiscal 1973. It is too early to assess the impact of the National
Health Services Corps on maldistribution. But the Health Services
Corps is an encouraging development and one in which physician's
assistants could play a role.

A DECLARATION OF LEGAL DEPENDENCE—
THE PA'S MAGNA CHARTA

By definition, the term "physician's assistant" signifies legal dependence. The success of the PA has been attributable in large part to a
close and legally dependent relationship to the traditional captain of
the health team, the physician.

The first PAs (1965—Duke version) were envisioned as
working alongside the physician wherever he went: hospital, operating room, office, clinic or patient's home. No other health professional does this. By remaining legally dependent to the physician, the
PA's range of activities is exceptionally broad. MDs can delegate to
PAs anything that they believe the PAs are competent to perform. As
they assume "associate" status, PAs perform an increasing array of
physician functions. They even resemble the physician in appearance
(short white coat with stethoscope, ophthalmoscope, etc.) and are
quickly surpassing other supporting health professionals in direct
patient management and in financial reward. In responsibility and
remuneration; they are coming to occupy the number two position
on the health team. Nursing, meanwhile, struggling for independence,
could well be outflanked by this "Johnny-come-lately" (see Chapter
Three, "Lessons from Nursing").

The implications of dependence and independence are
enormous and should be kept in mind throughout. Independence is
not necessarily an advantage for a profession or for patient care. An
alternative is interdependence which may solve some of the problems
posed by dependence and independence.[17] *Interdependence seems*

---

17. As Thelma Ingles, consultant in nursing for the Rockefeller
Foundation, has noted, the theme of interdependence has been expounded by
many nurses for some time. Objections to interdependence have come both from
organized nursing personnel who have demanded an independent role, and from
some physicians who advocate a dependent role.

to us to be the only rational solution if team care is to be a reality (see Chapter Five, "Organizational Alternatives"). The complexities of dependence vs. independence are also discussed in the legal section (see Chapter Four, "Where the Law Intervenes").

MALE AND FEMALE

In our view, it would be unfortunate to limit the physician's assistant profession to males, while other health professions, such as nursing, remain largely female. This is particularly important at a time when equal rights for the sexes are finally being recognized.

Nursing has traditionally been a profession for women. While little boys play soldier and doctor, little girls play mother and nurse. The very word "nurse" is sex-linked. The first definition of nurse in Webster's latest edition is "to nourish at the breast"—certainly not something men can provide.

The consequences for an all-female profession do not require much imagination. The nurse has been stuck with many of the thankless but vitally important nurturing and caring functions in the health system. For this she[18] has been underpaid, underutilized, and given little opportunity to advance to other fields. The recent emphasis on baccalaureate and graduate education for nurses has often helped to fan the fires of their frustration. Many nurses would rather stay at home and they do (see Chapter Three, "Lessons from Nursing").

Nowhere is her second class status more obvious than in the low pay she receives. An example from the medical literature is illuminating. The July 1969 issue of *Pediatrics* contained an article entitled "The Pediatric Nurse Practitioner in the Office of Pediatricians in Private Practice."[19] The authors were two pediatricians (part of a 10 man multispecialty group practice) and a pediatric nurse practitioner who worked for them. The article was filled with high praise for her excellent care and the outstanding patient acceptance of her work. A baccalaureate registered nurse and a graduate of Dr. Silver's Pediatric Nurse Practitioner Program, the article documented her ability to:

1. perform a total work-up of the well child (including complete physical examination),

---

18. The personal pronoun "she" will be used in relation to nursing because 99 percent of nurses are female.
19. Donald W. Schiff, Charles H. Fraser, and Heather L. Walters, "The Pediatric Nurse Practitioner in the Office of Pediatricians in Private Practice," *Pediatrics* 44, no. 1 (July 1969):62–68.

2. assist in the evaluation of sick patients,
3. counsel mothers on a large range of subjects,
4. coordinate activities of social workers and paramedical personnel,
5. give telephone advice to patients and decide when the physician is needed, and
6. perform and evaluate developmental and screening tests.

After an initial period of close supervision, she functioned increasingly independently with pediatrician backup limited to the unusual case. The office practice witnessed an increase of 18.8 percent over the number of patients previously seen by the two pediatricians combined. According to the article, she was so effective that "the physicians have not had to spend more time in the office, despite the increase in the number of patients seen."

For her outstanding labors she received a salary of $7,620 annually (37–46 percent greater than the salary of other registered nurses in the office!). Yet she netted an additional $16,800 for the office practice. (The authors were careful to point out that there has been no increase in overhead or space requirements.) They concluded that "the net income from charges made from the nurse's services exceeded the pediatric nurse practitioner's salary by the fifth month of her association with the office" and that *"having her in the office is an economic asset"* (emphasis added).

The salary discrimination by sex is buttressed by Dr. Silver's statement that many pediatric nurse practitioner graduates receive *no* increase in salary upon completion of their training.[20] *Graduates are still considered nurses first and pediatric practitioners second.* Discrimination by sex for nurse practitioners might be reduced if the name "nurse" were replaced by a neutral, nonfeminine title.

THE HIGH COST OF HEALTH CARE

Another explanation for the ability of the physician's assistant to surpass the nurse's income rests in the fundamental way in which health care is financed in this country. An examination of a relative fee schedule established in most states shows that the physician's fees are based on specific, discrete clinical services such as an appendectomy, a lumbar puncture, or the setting of a fracture. The equally important time invested in supportive patient management is not on the fee schedule and is not reimbursable.

---

20. Henry Silver—personal communication.

Typically, physician's assistants are paid a salary and do not receive directly the extra income generated for the physician's practice. If a physician charges physician rates for services performed by his assistant, he may benefit financially. If PAs are held to the same standard of care as the physician (as it appears they should be) then it is likely that the rates charged for those services will equal those of the physician. Will public and private health financing systems such as Medicare and Blue Cross be able to finance the costs of expanded care at physician rates?

Thus, the use of support personnel in physicians' offices may not save the consumer money. This is true whether the employee is male or female, physician's assistant or nurse. We do not think that consumers will tolerate this situation indefinitely as they watch medical bills soar out of sight.

However, the financing of health care is undergoing marked change in concert with the unmistakable trend toward the organized delivery of health services. In 1946, 404 groups of physicians practiced medicine in the United States. In 1969 the number increased to 6,371. This trend is irreversible in light of the increasing complexity of health care services. A projection is for 16,000 group practices by 1975.[21]

A 1971 amendment to the Social Security Act placed the federal government's purchasing power behind large health organizations referred to in the legislation as "health maintenance organizations." Under the social security amendments the health maintenance organization (HMO) is not paid by unit of service but is reimbursed by a lump sum prepaid contract.

The health maintenance organization has raised fundamental issues concerning the structure of the health care industry by fostering the evolution of large scale health care organizations which seek economies by offering a totality of services and benefits. Similarly, the HMO could affect the way in which the payment of salaries to physician's assistants and nurses is calculated. If salaries are based upon the efficiency with which health care (including maintenance and "caring") functions are delivered, there may be less tendency to base reimbursement on units of service rendered. The caring and maintenance functions should be more equitably reimbursable than today. And the consumer might be rewarded by less expensive health care.

In March 1972 Senator Edward Kennedy introduced the

21. Rick J. Carlson, "Health Manpower Licensing and Emerging Institutional Responsibility for the Quality of Care," *Law and Contemporary Problems* 35, no. 4 (Autumn 1970):849–78.

Health Maintenance Organization and Resources Development Act. The bill affirmed the administration's emphasis on the HMO as an essential new health care delivery mechanism but expanded greatly the scope of services to be provided.

National health insurance continues to be widely debated and strongly advocated by many political and professional leaders. Health leaders concerned with primary care and politicians interested in satisfying consumer needs may well identify the physician's assistant as a bulwark in the development of any national insurance scheme. Clearly, primary, emergency, and maintenance care should be cornerstone issues in any health insurance package. New and existing health professionals who are ostensibly able and willing to serve these important needs should occupy a major role in any national health insurance scheme.

Reimbursement for PA Services under Medicare

An early decision regarding payment for services under Medicare provided a serious challenge to the development of PAs. The issue initially stemmed from a May 10, 1971 letter from a Boston Bureau of Health Insurance official to a Medicare coordinator in New England. The letter stated: "The question of whether payment may be made for the services of physician's assistants who are physician employees depends . . . on whether they meet the requirements of Section 1861 (S)(2)(A) of the law which provides coverage of services 'furnished as incident to a physician's professional services of kinds which are commonly furnished in physician's offices and are commonly either rendered without charge or included in the physician's bills.' " It concluded that "Some of the services physician's assistants would perform would not presently meet the 'commonly furnished in physician's offices' requirement."

Naturally, this caused considerable concern among physician's assistant educators in New England. The concern was exacerbated when the Social Security Administration decided to adopt this interpretation as its national policy. In a September 28, 1971 letter to Senator Norris Cotton of New Hampshire, Mr. Robert M. Ball, Commissioner of Social Security, stated that "We have understood this provision of the law as intended by Congress to cover services of nurses and other assistants that are supportive to the physician's practice of medicine and are commonly furnished under his personal direction in his office." Commissioner Ball continued:

Accordingly, there are some services that Medex personnel perform in a physician's office which can be encompassed in the physician's service paid for under the Medicare program. These include various tasks that have been traditionally performed in physician's offices by nurses and aides; as for example, giving injections, performing blood tests, etc. Additionally, we believe that as the role of the physician's assistant in medical practice becomes established as professionally appropriate and acceptable, as well as consistent with state licensure, the Medicare program can take into account, for purposes of payment to a physician, a broader range of services by a physician's assistant, if they are commonly furnished in the physician's office and under his personal direction. Conversely, we would not construe to be covered under Medicare as 'incident to a physician's professional service' a medical procedure or act performed by a physician's assistant which takes on the character of independent practice—for example, a home call made by a Medex or, during an office visit, the treatment of a minor illness by the assistant, performed without involvement and review by the sponsoring physician. Any such extension of Medicare coverage would, we believe, have to occur as a result of legislative enactment and would have to specify what persons, under what conditions, and what amount could be reimbursed for the performance of such duties.

Thus, while one agency in HEW has given high priority to the funding of PA programs, another has denied reimbursement for many PA services.

Legislative change was forthcoming. On March 16, 1972 the Senate Finance Committee approved a modified version of an amendment offered by Senator Gaylord Nelson to HR 1. The amendment permits Medicare reimbursement for services performed by "assistants to physicians," both in and out of physician's offices, whether or not performed in the physician's presence. The committee agreed to allow HEW to conduct demonstration projects to determine the most appropriate and equitable levels of compensation. The committee modified the amendment to allow only experimental Medicare reimbursement for physician's assistants' services. The adoption of the amendment provided the flexibility needed for continuing experimental physician's assistant programs. With such a provision, the maximum utilization of PAs by physicians may be realized.

Support for Training the Physician's Assistant—Program Guidelines*

INTRODUCTION

Federal support for the training of physician's assistants responds to a number of forces, among them, the President's Health Message to Congress in 1971 and departmental policy. These, in turn, are based on goals for improved health care—access and availability, cost containment, and quality assurance. A growing consensus holds that simply producing more health workers will not counteract geographic and specialty maldistributions of manpower, nor will it constrain rapidly rising health care costs. Also required are more appropriate and efficient utilization of available skills, new types of health workers—especially the relatively scarce "midlevel" workers— and new working team relationships tied to health care delivery patterns in underserved areas.

The following policy guidelines are intended not as rigid standards, but as aids to the efficient and appropriately uniform achievement of the purposes for which the law was passed. Separate guidelines have been prepared for nurse practitioner programs.

SCOPE

Support for physician's assistant training through the Office of Special Programs, Bureau of Health Manpower Education, emphasizes preparation for primary ambulatory medical care in underserved areas. Such assistants would work with family physicians, internists,

---

*Taken from "Program Support for Physician's Assistants in Primary Care," March 1972, prepared by U.S. Department of Health, Education and Welfare, Bureau of Health Manpower Education, Office of Special Programs.

pediatricians, obstetricians, and in outpatient and emergency care facilities. Programs with a more limited specialty orientation (such as urology or orthopedics) should apply for grant support under authorities of the Division of Allied Health Manpower, 9000 Rockville Pike, Bethesda, Maryland 20014.

DEFINITION—PHYSICIAN'S ASSISTANT

The term physician's assistant, as used for purposes of program administration, refers to one who by training and experience is prepared to work under the supervision of a licensed physician to aid that physician in carrying out his patient care responsibilities. The physician's assistant is prepared to collect a "data base" through a medical history, general physical examination and routine laboratory tests, to organize the information to aid the physician in diagnosis, and to administer treatments as prescribed by the physician. He may, on the basis of standing orders, treat a defined range of medical conditions and may provide emergency care in keeping with his training and as permitted by his supervising physician. Although effective supervision is required, it need not in all cases be face to face.

The assistant may be prepared and permitted to perform other technical or clinical tasks—laboratory, X-ray, etc.—as determined by the training program and the individual supervising physician.

EDUCATION AND TRAINING

All programs should meet the "Minimum Essentials, Physician's Assistant—Generalist," of the Council on Medical Education, American Medical Association.

Applicants for training support may be medical centers having appropriate educational resources or support, medical schools, health science centers, and academic settings, primarily schools of allied health professions.

RECRUITMENT OF STUDENTS

Priority for support will be given to those programs which build on previous training and experience (including military) and/or which recruit from underserved areas those persons most likely to secure appropriate employment and remain in those areas.

GENERAL CONSIDERATIONS

Programs will be supported only in those states where the employment of such assistants is not in violation of the state's medical practice act.

Practicing primary care physicians, either as individuals or groups, should be actively involved with the program.

Programs must demonstrate a relationship to an underserved area and must provide reasonable assurance that graduates can actually be employed in such areas.

Because of the provisional nature of the work-role of the physician's assistant, programs should assume responsibility for follow-up of graduates both as a check on the validity of their educational program and to assure realistic clinical competency based on employment requirements.

SUPPORT

Support for training programs will be primarily through the contract method. Although contracts must be reviewed and negotiated annually, support for a three to five year period is anticipated.

For purposes of cost comparison and control in establishing support priorities, the total budget should be broken into the following categories:

1. start-up costs (for new programs only),
2. instructional costs (including program evaluation),
3. student support (only where absolutely essential), and
4. follow-up of graduate performance (optional).

A "cost per graduate" will be computed as one factor in establishing funding priorities.

Resource Document

Essentials of an Approved Educational Program for the Assistant to the Primary Care Physician*

OBJECTIVE

The education and health professions cooperate in this program to establish and maintain standards of appropriate quality for educational programs for the assistant to the primary care physician, and to provide recognition for educational programs which meet or exceed the minimal standards outlined in these essentials.

These standards are to be used as a guide for the development and self-evaluation of programs for the assistant to the primary care physician. Lists of these approved programs are published for the information of employers and the public. Students enrolled in the programs are taught to work with and under the direction of physicians in providing health care services to patients.

DESCRIPTION OF THE OCCUPATION

The assistant to the primary care physician is a skilled person, qualified by academic and clinical training to provide patient services under the supervision and responsibility of a doctor of medicine or osteopathy who is, in turn, responsible for the performance of that assistant. The assistant may be involved with the patients of the physician in any medical setting for which the physician is responsible.

---

*Prepared by the American Medical Association Council on Medical Education, in collaboration with the American Academy of Family Physicians, the American Academy of Pediatrics, the American College of Physicians, and the American Society of Internal Medicine. Adopted by the AMA House of Delegates, December 1971. "Assistant to the primary care physician" is a generic term.

The function of the assistant to the primary care physician is to perform, under the responsibility and supervision of the physician, diagnostic and therapeutic tasks in order to allow the physician to extend his services through the more effective use of his knowledge, skills, and abilities.

In rendering services to his patients, the primary care physician is traditionally involved in a variety of activities. Some of these activities, including the application of his knowledge toward a logical and systematic evaluation of the patient's problems and planning a program of management and therapy appropriate to the patient, can only be performed by the physician. The assistant to the primary care physician will not supplant the doctor in the sphere of the decisionmaking required to establish a diagnosis and plan therapy, but will assist in gathering the data necessary to reach decisions and in implementing the therapeutic plan for the patient.

Intelligence, the ability to relate to people, a capacity for calm and reasoned judgment in meeting emergencies, and an orientation toward service are qualities essential for the assistant to the primary care physician. As a professional, he must maintain respect for the person and privacy of the patient.

The tasks performed by the assistant will include transmission and execution of physician's orders, performance of patient care tasks, and performance of diagnostic and therapeutic procedures as may be delegated by the physician.

Since the function of the primary care physician is interdisciplinary in nature, involving the five major clinical disciplines (medicine, surgery, pediatrics, psychiatry, and obstetrics) within the limitations and capabilities of the particular practice in consideration, the assistant to the primary care physician should be involved in assisting the physician provide those varied medical services necessary for the total health care of the patient.

The ultimate role of the assistant to the primary care physician cannot be rigidly defined because of the variations in practice requirements due to geographic, economic, and sociologic factors. The high degree of responsibility an assistant to the primary care physician may assume requires that, at the conclusion of his formal education, he possess the knowledge, skills, and abilities necessary to provide those services appropriate to the primary care setting. These services would include, but need not be limited to, the following:

1. the initial approach to a patient of any age group in any setting to elicit a detailed and accurate history, perform an appropriate

physical examination, and record and present pertinent data in a manner meaningful to the physician;

2. performance and/or assistance in performance of routine laboratory and related studies as appropriate for a specific practice setting, such as the drawing of blood samples, performance of urinalyses, and the taking of electrocardiographic tracings;
3. performance of such routine therapeutic procedures as injections, immunizations, and the suturing and care of wounds;
4. instruction and counseling of patients regarding physical and mental health on matters such as diets, disease, therapy, and normal growth and development;
5. assisting the physician in the hospital setting by making patient rounds, recording patient progress notes, accurately and appropriately transcribing and/or executing standing orders and other specific orders at the direction of the supervising physician, and compiling and recording detailed narrative case summaries;
6. providing assistance in the delivery of services to patients requiring continuing care (home, nursing home, extended care facilities, etc.) including the review and monitoring of treatment and therapy plans;
7. independent performance of evaluative and treatment procedures essential to provide an appropriate response to life-threatening, emergency situations; and
8. facilitation of the physician's referral of appropriate patients by maintenance of an awareness of the community's various health facilities, agencies, and resources.

ESSENTIAL REQUIREMENTS

I. *Educational Programs May Be Established in*

A. medical schools,
B. senior colleges and universities in affiliation with an accredited teaching hospital;
C. medical educational facilities of the federal government; and
D. other institutions with clinical facilities, which are acceptable to the Council on Medical Education of the American Medical Association.

The institution should be accredited or otherwise acceptable to the Council on Medical Education. Senior colleges and universities must have the necessary clinical affiliations.

II. Clinical Affiliations

A. The clinical phase of the educational program must be conducted in a clinical setting and under competent clinical direction.

B. In programs where the academic instruction and clinical teaching are not provided in the same institution, accreditation shall be given to the institution responsible for the academic preparation (student selection, curriculum, academic credit, etc.) and the educational administrators shall be responsible for assuring that the activities assigned to students in the clinical setting are, in fact, educational.

C. In the clinical teaching environment, an appropriate ratio of students to physicians shall be maintained.

III. Facilities

A. Adequate classrooms, laboratories, and administrative offices should be provided.

B. Appropriate modern equipment and supplies for directed experience should be available in sufficient quantities.

C. A library should be readily accessible and should contain an adequate supply of up to date, scientific books, periodicals, and other reference materials related to the curriculum.

IV. Finances

A. Financial resources for continued operation of the educational program shall be assured for each class of students enrolled.

B. The institution shall not charge excessive student fees.

C. Advertising must be appropriate to an educational institution.

D. The program shall not substitute students for paid personnel to conduct the work of the clinical facility.

V. Faculty

A. Program Director
   1. The program director should meet the requirements specified by the institution providing the didactic portion of the educational program.
   2. The program director should be responsible for the organization, administration, periodic review, continued development, and general effectiveness of the program.

B. Medical Director
   1. The medical director should provide competent medical direction for the clinical instruction and for clinical relationships with other educational programs. He should have the understanding and support of practicing physicians.

2. The medical director should be a physician experienced in the delivery of the type of health care services for which the student is being trained.

3. The medical director may also be the program director.

C. Change of Director
If the program director or medical director is changed, immediate notification should be sent to the AMA Department of Allied Medical Professions and Services. The curriculum vitae of the new director, giving details of his training, education, and experience, must be submitted.

D. Instructional Staff
1. The faculty must be qualified, through academic preparation and experience, to teach the subjects assigned.
2. The faculty for the clinical portion of the educational program must include physicians who are involved in the provision of patient care services. Because of the unique characteristics of the assistant to the primary care physician, it is necessary that the preponderance of clinical teaching be conducted by practicing physicians.

E. Advisory Committee
An advisory committee should be appointed to assist the director in continuing program development and evaluation, in faculty coordination, and in coordination of effective clinical relationships. For maximum effectiveness, an advisory committee should include representation of the primary institution involved, the program administration, organized medicine, the practicing physician, and others.

VI. Students

A. Selection
1. Selection of students should be made by an admissions committee in cooperation with those responsible for the educational program. Admissions data should be on file at all times in the institution responsible for the administration of the program.
2. Selection procedures must include an analysis of previous performance and experience and may seek to accommodate candidates with a health-related background and give due credit for the knowledge, skills, and abilities they possess.

B. Health
Applicants shall be required to submit evidence of good health. When students are learning in a clinical setting or a hospital, the hospital or clinical setting should provide them with the protec-

tion of the same physical examinations and immunizations as are provided to hospital employees working in the same clinical setting.

C. Number
The number of students enrolled in each class should be commensurate with the most effective learning and teaching practices and should also be consistent with acceptable student-teacher ratios.

D. Counseling
A student guidance and placement service should be available.

E. Student Identification
Students enrolled in the educational program must be clearly identified to distinguish them from physicians, medical students, and students and personnel for other health occupations.

VII. Records

Satisfactory records should be provided for all work accomplished by the student while enrolled in the program. Annual reports of the operation of the program should be prepared and available for review.

A. Student
1. Transcripts of high school and any college credits and other credentials must be on file.
2. Reports of medical examination upon admission and records of any subsequent illness during training should be maintained.
3. Records of class and laboratory participation and academic and clinical achievements of each student should be maintained in accordance with the requirements of the institution.

B. Curriculum
1. A synopsis of the current curriculum should be kept on file.
2. This synopsis should include the rotation of assignments, the outline of the instruction supplied, and lists of multimedia instructional aids used to augment the experience of the student.

C. Activity
1. A satisfactory record system shall be provided for all student performance.
2. Practical and written examinations should be continually evaluated.

VIII. *Curriculum*

A. The length of the educational program for the assistant to the primary care physician may vary from program to program. The length of time an individual spends in the training program may vary on the basis of the student's background and in consideration of his previous education, experience, knowledge, skills, and abilities, and his ability to perform the tasks, functions, and duties implied in the "Description of the Occupation."

B. Instruction, tailored to meet the student's needs, should follow a planned outline including:
   1. assignment of appropriate instructional materials;
   2. classroom presentations, discussions, and demonstrations;
   3. supervised practice discussions; and
   4. examinations, tests, and quizzes—both practical and written—for the didactic and clinical portions of the educational program.

C. General courses or topics of study, both didactic and clinical, should include the following:
   1. The general courses and topics of study must be achievement-oriented and provide the graduates with the necessary knowledge, skills, and abilities to accurately and reliably perform the tasks, functions, and duties implied in the "Description of the Occupation."
   2. Instruction should be sufficiently comprehensive so as to provide the graduate with an understanding of mental and physical disease in both the ambulatory and hospitalized patient. Attention should also be given to preventive medicine and public health and to the social and economic aspects of the systems for delivering health and medical services. Instruction should stress the role of the assistant to the primary care physician relative to the health maintenance and medical care of his supervising physician's patients. Throughout, the student should be encouraged to develop those basic intellectual, ethical, and moral attitudes and principles that are essential for his gaining and maintaining the trust of those with whom he works and the support of the community in which he lives.
   3. A "model unit of primary medical care," such as the models used in departments of family practice in medical schools and family practice residencies, should be encouraged so that the

medical student, the resident, and the assistant to the primary care physician can jointly share the educational experience in an atmosphere that reflects and encourages the actual practice of primary medical care.

4. The curriculum should be broad enough to provide the assistant to the primary care physician with the technical capabilities, behavioral characteristics, and judgment necessary to perform in a professional capacity all of his assignments, and should take into consideration any proficiency and knowledge obtained elsewhere and demonstrated prior to completion of the program.

IX. Administration

A. An official publication, including a description of the program, should be available. It should include information regarding the organization of the program, a brief description of required courses, names and academic rank of faculty, entrance requirements, tuition and fees, and information concerning hospitals and facilities used for training.

B. The evaluation (including survey team visits) of a program of study must be initiated by the express invitation of the chief administrator of the institution or his officially designated representative.

C. The program may withdraw its request for initial approval at any time (even after evaluation) prior to final action. The AMA Council on Medical Education and the collaborating organizations may withdraw approval whenever:

1. the educational program is not maintained in accordance with the standards outlined above, or
2. there are no students in the program for two consecutive years.

Approval is withdrawn only after advance notice has been given to the director of the program that such action is contemplated, and the reasons therefore, sufficient to permit timely response and use of the established procedure for appeal and review.

D. Evaluation
1. The head of the institution being evaluated is given an opportunity to become acquainted with the factual part of the report prepared by the visiting survey team, and to comment on its accuracy before final action is taken.
2. At the request of the head of the institution, a reevaluation may be made. Adverse decisions may be appealed in writing

to the Council on Medical Education of the American Medical Association.

E. Reports

An annual report should be made to the AMA Council on Medical Education and the collaborating organizations. A report form is provided and should be completed, signed by the program director, and returned promptly.

F. Reevaluation

The American Medical Association and collaborating organizations will periodically reevaluate and provide consultation to educational programs.

X. Changes in Essentials

Proposed changes in the "Essentials of an Approved Educational Program for the Assistant to the Primary Care Physician" will be considered by a standing committee representing the spectrum of approved programs for the assistant to the primary care physician, the American Academy of Family Physicians, the American Academy of Pediatrics, the American College of Physicians, and the American Society of Internal Medicine. Recommended changes will be submitted to these collaborating organizations and the American Medical Association.

XI. Applications and Inquiries

Applications for program approval should be directed to:

Department of Allied Medical Professions and Services
Division of Medical Education
American Medical Association
535 North Dearborn Street
Chicago, Illinois 60610

Chapter Three

Lessons from Nursing

NURSING UPSTAGED?

The appearance of the physician's assistant on the health manpower stage has been greeted by most critics with rave notices but has been panned by others. Many puzzle about how the physician's assistant was written into the script rather than the nurse who seems the more logical choice, being a known quantity to both patients and physicians who have been assisted greatly by her caring help over the years.

There are several cogent reasons for looking at nursing in the belief that it will inform the future of the physician's assistant. Not the least is the question of why medicine created the new health category of physician's assistant rather than seek to expand the nurse's role. Nursing, in fact, was approached by the AMA late in 1969 and invited to play an expanded role as a physician's assistant. The AMA offer was met with such rebuff that medicine then focused its attentions on the non-nurse physician's assistant.

There are other reasons that the physician's assistant movement can learn a great deal from nursing. For one, the development of the physician's assistant shares certain historical parallels with nursing. Nurses traditionally have rendered care to patients in a dependent relationship with physicians. The push of late for what nursing calls independence may really be a quest for clearer professional identity. In this connection, the evolution of professionalism in nursing has an interesting history which may presage the efforts of the physician's assistant movement to professionalize itself. Yet, wedded as both the nurse and physician's assistant are to the physician, there is still a great unidentified potential for interface between traditional nursing at all levels and the physician's assistant. In situations where nurses work side by side with PAs in *legally dependent* relationship to a physician, some of their functions will overlap as the boundaries among these three health professions become less distinct. Their work together cannot help but stimulate redefinitions of roles among nurses, physician's assistants, and physicians as they form *interdependent* relationships on behalf of improved patient care.

It is also important in considering the future of the physician's assistant movement to take into account reactions of the nursing profession. From its inception in 1965, the physician's assistant concept captured nursing's interest. Nursing has taken an increasingly active role in examining the present status and future thrust of the physician's assistant vis-à-vis nursing. There is no doubt that nursing intends to have its say. There is a growing body of nursing literature in which the profession's leaders address the PA issue.[1]

In addition, several groups have issued official policy statements about the physician's assistant which reflect the nursing profession's concerns about the concept.[2] Chief among the stated concerns are the questionable need for the PA, lack of universally accepted guidelines for use of PAs in the health care system, comparable salaries, and the carrying out of physician's assistant orders by the nurse.

Hence, any examination of the development of the physician's assistant concept without consideration of the nursing profession would be found wanting. Likewise, any examination of the present status and future thrust of nursing, without due considera-

---

1. Foremost among them: Dorothy Mereness, "Recent Trends in Expanding Roles of the Nurse," *Nursing Outlook* 18, no. 5 (May 1970):30–33; Ava Dilworth, "Joint Preparation for Clinical Nurse Specialists," *Nursing Outlook* 18, no. 9 (September 1970):22–25; Eleanor C. Lambertsen, "Nursing: Not Quite M.D., More Than P.A.," *Hospitals, JAHA* 45: no. 23 (December 1, 1971):70–76; Martha E. Rogers, "Nursing: To Be or Not To Be?" *Nursing Outlook* 20, no. 1 (January 1972):42–46.
2. National Commission for the Study of Nursing and Nursing Education, "Nurse Clinician and Physician's Assistant: The Relationship Between Two Emerging Practitioner Concepts" (Lysaught commission brochure, 1970), (see pp. 65–76); Massachusetts Nurses Association, "Position Statement on the Physician's Assistant" (March 1971), (see pp. 81–82); American Nurses Association, "The American Nurses Association Views The Emerging Physician's Assistant" (December 21, 1971), (see pp. 77–79); New York State Nurses Association, "Statement on the Physician's Associate and Specialist's Assistant" (January 31, 1972), (see pp. 83–85).
The physician's assistant has also been considered by the AMA–ANA National Joint Practice Commission.

tion of the physician's assistant movement, is wishful thinking and may result in premature closure in two professions which need more than anything else *interdependent* relationships on behalf of improved patient care.

NURSING TODAY: DIVERSITY, SCHISM, FLIGHT, AND FIGHT

The nation's greatly improved level of health in this century has been enhanced enormously by the contributions of the nursing profession. However, along with much that is good, there are some unfortunate developments within organized nursing which threaten to diminish nursing's future contributions to a nation in search of better health.

Four characteristics problematic to the profession of nursing today provide a scaffolding from which to view with hindsight centenarian nursing and to plan with foresight the future of the physician's assistant, as yet a stripling.

Diversity

Nursing is a diverse health profession with numerous levels of knowledge, skills, and responsibilities. These levels range from the "technical" level of nurses aide, licensed practical nurse, associate degree, and diploma nurse, through the "professional" levels beginning with a baccalaureate nurse and the nonmaster's nurse practitioner to the more sophisticated master's nurse clinician and finally the nurse with a doctorate or Ph.D (see Figure 3–1). The term "nurse," like the term "physician's assistant," has become so general that, in speaking of the nurse, it is necessary to specify the level intended.

At the base of the nursing education pyramid are the aides, orderlies, and attendants who are trained on the job over a period of months in the employing hospital. The licensed practical nurse is trained by the hospital nursing service in one year. Diploma nurses receive three years of training with heavy emphasis on clinical experience rather than theory. Associate degree nurses receive a junior college education combined with limited clinical exposure. However, the associate degree nurse has the advantage of being on the education ladder.

The baccalaureate nurse graduates at the end of four academic years in college as a beginning practitioner. Two of her four years concentrate on liberal arts. The remaining two years of credit are earned in nursing theory and brief periods of clinical experience. Clinical specialization or teaching credentials are acquired

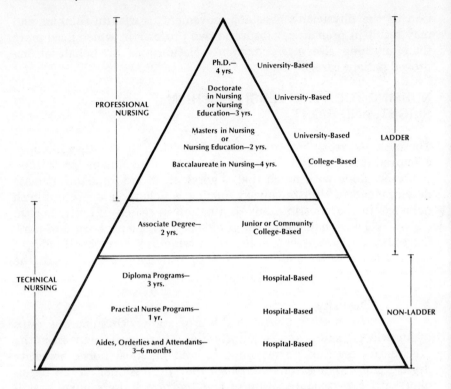

Figure 3–1. The Nursing Education Pyramid

at the master's or higher degree level. Even these programs have less clinical practice than similar higher degree programs in social work, psychology, teaching, or medicine.

There is great disparity between educational levels and the clinical component of nurse preparation. The least educated registered nurse from the diploma program receives the greatest amount of clinical preparation while the more educated baccalaureate nurse receives much less. Nursing educators quickly point out that quantity is not to be confused with quality and that one good hour of learning in a baccalaureate program is worth ten hours of mindless service in a diploma program. Yet the lack of clinical experience in college-based nursing programs is such a problem that a study of why 66 baccalaureate nursing students sought paid part time and summer nursing jobs found that they *all* did so primarily to gain clinical experience in nursing and gain self-confidence in their nursing skills.[3]

---

3. Mary Louise Paynich, "Why Do Basic Nursing Students Work in Nursing?," *Nursing Outlook* 19, no. 4 (April 1971):242–45.

Table 3–1. Practicing Professional and Technical Nurses—A Decade
of Supply and Demand

	1962 Supply[1]	1967 Supply[2]	1972 Supply[3]
Professional Nurses			
Master's or higher	11,500	16,000	19,000[4]
baccalaureate	43,500	67,600	80,000
Technical Nurses			
Diploma	495,000	556,400	579,000
Associate degree	—	—	22,000
Total	550,000	640,000	700,000

1. HEW Public Health Service. Report of the Surgeon General's Consultant Group on Nursing, *Toward Quality in Nursing* (1963), ch. IV, "Needs for 1970," pp. 15–19.
2. HEW Bureau of Health Manpower, Division of Nursing, *Nurse Training Act of 1964 Program Review Report* (December 1967), figure 3, p. 57.
3. American Nurses Association, Department of Research and Statistics (March 1972).
4. Less than 700 Ph.D. or doctorate.

Schism Between Nursing Education and Service

There is a paradoxical schism in nursing today between nursing education and nursing service. A master's or higher degree is the minimal ticket of admission to teaching. Of the 700,000 practicing nurses in 1972, fewer than 20,000 (3 percent) held a master's degree or higher. Yet the nursing educators tend to be the spokesmen for the profession while direct patient care is given by the nearly 600,000 diploma nurses (see Table 3–1).

In other words, nursing *educators*, with their commitment to baccalaureate and higher education, constitute 3 percent of the practicing profession but determine educational policy for the other 97 percent who provide the *service*. This split within nursing has been cited by Ginzberg as a high hurdle to moving readily to new goals and objectives.[4] The need for closer ties between nursing education and nursing service has been frequently voiced.[5]

4. Eli Ginzberg, *Men, Money and Medicine* (New York: Columbia University Press, 1969), p. 166.
5. HEW Bureau of Health Manpower, Division of Nursing, *Nurse Training Act of 1964 Program Review Report* (December 1967), p. 24; National Commission for the Study of Nursing and Nursing Education, *An Abstract for Action* (New York: McGraw-Hill, 1970), pp. 28–32, 94–96; Janelle C. Krueger, "The Education and Utilization of Nurses: A Paradox," *Nursing Outlook* 19, no. 10 (October 1971):676–79.

Flight

Nursing education struggles to replace diploma nurses with steadily increasing numbers of baccalaureate and master's graduates whose impact on service is mitigated by their flight from hospital work. As will be elaborated upon later, the disappointment experienced by baccalaureate graduates often is born of false expectations engendered during their education which dissipate into hopelessness in the reality of hospital practice.

Fight

There has been strife between organized nursing and organized medicine which has greatly impeded their ability to work together to improve patient care. This has been compounded by the lack of cohesiveness within nursing itself.

Because we wish a safer crossing into professionalism for the physician's assistant, a careful look into how nursing arrived at its present state seems warranted. We are certain that valuable lessons for the physician's assistant lie between the lines which follow.

NURSING EDUCATION:
BUILDING BLOCKS FOR THE SIXTIES;
STUMBLING BLOCKS FOR THE SEVENTIES?

How did nursing education gain dominant influence in the nursing profession? The beginning of college education of nurses goes back to the 1920s but it was not until the 1960s that nursing education firmly rooted itself in higher education. The reasons for this are enmeshed in the values of that decade.

The sixties witnessed a nation's dedication to education. Both the nation's dreams and resources were heaped upon educational institutions in pursuit of an increase in the quantity and quality of education. The ultimate birthright was seen as education through college for every capable young American regardless of color or class. It was an auspicious climate for the profession of nursing to consolidate its position in the university and to secure a snug harbor in academe.

The building blocks for nursing in the sixties rest upon four historic documents in the profession which greatly reflect the educational priorities of their time:

1. Report of the Surgeon General's Consultant Group on Nursing, 1963;
2. Nurse Training Act of 1964, Public Law 88–581;

3. ANA position paper, "Educational Preparation for Nurse Practitioners and Assistants to Nurses," 1965;
4. National Commission for the Study of Nursing and Nursing Education, 1969.

The Surgeon General's report of 1963 forecast nursing's subsequent commitment to higher education: "[We are] convinced that the baccalaureate program should be the minimal requirement for nurses who will assume leadership."[6] A break with entrenched patterns in nursing education was suggested. As a note of caution, however, precipitous change was eschewed in favor of an orderly transition from hospital-based training resources to colleges and universities.

Also urged was a broad, comprehensive study, perhaps requiring five to ten years, of "basic nursing education in relation to the responsibilities and skill levels required for high-quality patient care."[7] And, as is common to such reports, the final plea was one for federal funds to schools of nursing to improve their educational programs, and to colleges to entice them to establish new schools of nursing.[8]

Response to the Surgeon General's report was rapid and committed. Congress enacted the Nurse Training Act of 1964 which provided the money to carry out the suggested enhancement of nursing education. Construction of facilities, expanded programs, and loans and traineeships to nursing students flourished under this legislation.

In 1965, the American Nurses' Association (ANA) prepared a position paper which divided nurses into two categories, depending upon educational preparation:

1. *Professional Nurses* for whom minimum preparation for beginning professional nursing should be baccalaureate degree education in nursing;[9] and
2. *Technical Nurses* for whom minimum preparation for beginning technical nursing practice should be associate degree education in nursing.[10]

---

6. HEW Public Health Service, Report of the Surgeon General's Consultant Group on Nursing, *Toward Quality in Nursing* (1963), ch. IV, "Needs for 1970," pp. 15–19.
7. Ibid., p. 34.
8. Ibid., p. 56.
9. American Nurses Association Position Paper, "Educational Preparation for Nurse Practitioners and Assistants to Nurses" (1965), p. 6 (see pp. 57–63).
10. Ibid., p. 8.

The final building block of the decade for nursing education was *An Abstract for Action*, also known as the Lysaught report, written by the National Commission for the Study of Nursing Education, and funded by the Kellogg and Avalon Foundations, the ANA, and an anonymous donor.[11] The Lysaught report was the result of a three year study, including:

- twelve commissioners;
- a director, an associate director, and their staff of seven;
- four advisory panels totaling 34 members;
- 139 representatives of health professions who made their contributions in over a dozen regional conferences; and
- more than 1,000 nurses, physicians, administrators, researchers, students, and consumers interviewed during 100 site visits throughout the United States.

The commission's charge was to "illuminate the characteristics, concepts, and scope of nursing practice." The report focused instead on how to reorganize nursing to enable it to communicate and work with other health professions, especially medicine. Had the commission more adequately studied the present system of nursing education in relation to responsibilities and skill levels, its report would have constituted nursing's homework for the interdisciplinary national and state joint practice commissions which it subsequently recommended and which was the organizational crux of the entire report. A substantive definition of nursing's "responsibilities and skill levels" would have buttressed.nursing's position as it met with other disciplines, and the Lysaught report could have become more of a working paper and less of an organizational document in search of funding.

In summary, the surgeon general's report of 1963 provided impetus to nursing education; the Nurse Training Act of 1964 gave it the wherewithal; the ANA position paper of 1965 endowed nursing with a philosophy for future direction, which the Lysaught report sought to augment.

Building Blocks into Stumbling Blocks?

What were building blocks for nursing in the sixties may be its stumbling blocks in the seventies as it faces the new challenge to provide more health care. Indeed, one unfortunate outcome of the

---

11. National Commission for the Study of Nursing and Nursing Education, *An Abstract for Action*.

academizing of the nursing profession has been its isolation from the realities of service. The reasons for this schism between nursing education and service deserve both understanding and sympathy.

When in 1971 a patient care institution as venerable as Massachusetts General Hospital suffers a 64 percent turnover[12] of baccalaureate, diploma, and associate degree nursing staff and the New York City hospitals a turnover rate of 86 percent,[13] something is seriously wrong. Among those things wrong are the nurse misused and the nurse abused.

The Nurse Misused

Why teach the nurse anatomy, physiology, chemistry, anthropology, microbiology, the signs and symptoms of disease, the course of and response to medications, and other therapeutic procedures, as well as the possible outcome and complications, if she is unable to utilize this information in ways which directly improve the patient's health? If the nurse, as suggested by some, should only collect data and make observations, then a brief course in interviewing is all that is needed. Why teach pharmacology now that the pharmacy in many hospitals prepares the proper dosages in separate packages and the nurse may only deliver them to the patient? Why take the long time to fill the nurse's head with signs and symptoms of disease if diagnosis is not to be her function? To what avail physiology and anatomy if the nurse may only sponge it, roll it over, or assist it out of bed?

If the nurse is to offer primarily succor and tender loving care rendered with dignity, then the education of nurses could be greatly simplified and shortened. Merely screen for poised young women who show sensitivity to others and are of naturally pleasant disposition. Then teach them in short order the basics of observation, data collection, body care, comfort measures, and emphasize therapeutic interaction with others. The time to prepare such a nurse should take little more than six months and as such resembles the training of the licensed practical nurse or nurses' aide! The alternative to this, of course, is to continue to educate nurses in the basic sciences and pathology, give them breadth and depth of clinical experience, but use them to full benefit of the many patients who can be helped by the nurse's knowledge and skills.

---

12. Mary MacDonald, Director, Department of Nursing, Massachusetts General Hospital (personal communication). This was a 14 percent reduction from the 1968 turnover of 78 percent. A vigorous inservice program instituted since 1968 has been given credit for the reduction in turnover.
13. "City Hospitals Struggle With Nursing Shortage," *New York Times*, April 23, 1971, pp. 39, 46.

The Nurse Abused

There are over half a million nurses in the country who choose not to practice their profession! (see Figure 3-2).

Not only is the rate of inactivity disturbing evidence of trouble within the profession, but nurses display a greater rate of turnover in their profession than women with similar education and training in most other professions. As documented by the Lysaught commission's *An Abstract for Action* and its brochure "Nurse Clinician and Physician's Assistant," the average rate of turnover among staff nurses in American hospitals is over 70 percent while the rate of turnover among elementary and secondary school teachers—also predominantly female and from the same socioeconomic backgrounds—is approximately 20 percent.

Some of the problems responsible for the turnover and dropping out of nurses have been identified as lack of direct patient care by nurses who are siphoned off into managerial functions of overseeing the care provided by others; poor compensation; and unsatisfactory working hours. What other professional of similar educational preparation is required to work all shifts within one week as is the lot of many nurses? Management research has found that while money and working conditions such as hours are job dissatisfiers, they are not satisfiers. Herzberg pursues in detail job

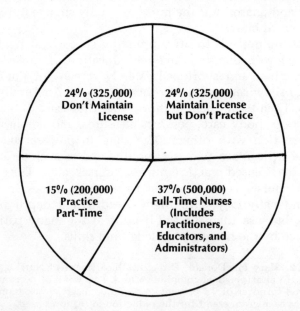

Figure 3-2. Distribution of Activity Among Graduate Nurses

satisfiers versus dissatisfiers and clusters chief job satisfiers around self-esteem.[14] The need for self-esteem also looms paramount in Maslow's hierarchy of needs. Given the importance of self-esteem in job satisfaction, the nurse's unmet needs for recognition and self-esteem are critical.[15]

As long ago as 1961, Bennis concluded from his research of nurses in the outpatient department and his review of studies by others: "We see that there is almost no situation presently available to the graduate nurse which will allow her to perform according to the traditional conception of the ideal nursing role. This is clearly an intolerable situation for a professional, and definite remedial steps need be taken. Either practice situations will have to be transformed to fit into the concept currently being taught in educational institutions or the concept will have to be changed to more appropriately reflect practice."[16]

Yet ten years later, in 1971, Golub described the plight of the new baccalaureate graduates who experienced a gap between expectations and nursing service demands: "The end results of the plight of the new graduate should be of concern to all. Studies have shown that the new nurse often quits her first hospital job within the first year (or *never* chooses hospital nursing) or soon loses any ideals or commitments or emulates the status quo even to the point of developing bad nursing habits." Golub also scored the "inability of nursing service to define clearly what nursing areas are; to test out, utilize, or add to theories and studies of nursing science and education; or to agree on what is expected of its own nursing practitioners."[17]

Many of these problems can be attributed to physicians and hospital administrators, as well as to nurses. A study by Krueger of the activities of 128 baccalaureate, diploma, practical nurses, and aides pointed to a gap between the "ideal" use of the nurse taught by education and their "real" use by employers.[18]

It has been the universities which have endowed nursing with a respectability, freedom, and responsibility which embody the

---

14. Frederick Herzberg, Bernard Mausner, and Barbara Snyderman, *The Motivation to Work* (New York: John Wiley and Sons, 1959).
15. Abraham Maslow, *Motivation and Personality*, 2nd ed. (New York: Harper and Row, 1970), ch. 4.
16. Warren Bennis, Norman Berkowitz, Mary Malone, and Malcolm Klein, *The Role of the Nurse in the Out-Patient Department* (New York: American Nurses' Foundation, 1961), p. 63.
17. Judith Golub, "A Nurse-Internship Program," *Hospitals, JAHA* 45 (August 16, 1971):73–78.
18. Krueger, pp. 676–79.

self-esteem that nursing has not been able to enjoy in the hospital sickroom despite a century of service. Whereas nurses have suffered misuse and abuse in service settings, they have been welcomed by the academicians with the only requirement that nurses join scholars in the pursuit of excellence of scholarship in an atmosphere of free and systematic inquiry. Unfortunately, the discrepancy between what the baccalaureate nurse is taught about ideal patient care in the university and the reality demands of hospital settings today too often leads her to a profound personal crisis which is resolved more often by flight than fight. This is unlike the preparation of the diploma nurse whose knowledge and procedural skills are molded in the image of hospital practice so that upon graduation the nurse hardly breaks step in making the transition from student to hospital staff nurse.

Diploma nurses who render the majority of care in hospitals find it difficult to move out of hospitals because they lack the baccalaureate degree deemed essential by organized nursing to practice in a greater variety of settings such as public health, teaching, or school nursing. Organized nursing neither favors nor facilitates the diploma nurse acquiring the necessary college education beyond her nursing skills, preferring instead the unadulterated socialization process of molding the college undergraduate into its ideal of the thinking, empathic nurse with minimal procedural skills.

The 1965 ANA Position Paper: A Bias Without Basis?

The increases in college-based programs since 1964 reflect in large part the financial boost received from the Nurse Training Act of that year which provided bricks and mortar, traineeships for students, incentive grants for faculty, and curricular innovations for the collegiate programs. However, the burgeoning of baccalaureate programs clearly owes its impetus to the ANA 1965 position paper, which stated unequivocally that the education for all those licensed to practice nursing should take place in institutions of higher education.

The ANA decision to prepare nurses in institutions of higher learning has resulted in a significant decline in diploma programs accompanied by a steady increase in baccalaureate and a rapid rise in associate degree programs (see Table 3-2.)

In the foreword to their position paper, the ANA claims to have undertaken "the study and examination of nursing education, the nature and characteristics of nursing practice, and the scope of preparation and responsibilities of nurses." After two years of study, the ANA Committee on Education put forth an array of assumptions

Table 3–2. Trends in Nursing Education by Type of Program,
1952 to 1972

Type of Program	1952	1962	1972
Nurse scientist			9
Ph.D. or doctorate		4	8
Master's		48	79
Baccalaureate degree	198	176	290
Diploma	1017	875	550
Associate degree	21	84	485
Total Programs	1236	1187	1421

apparently more philosophically than scientifically derived, from which their position issued. The composition of the ANA Committee on Education, all nurse educators with rank of dean, suggests a bias toward collegiate education. Nursing service leaders were conspicuous by their absence. Central to the controversy about hospital-based versus college-based programs is the quality of the prepared student.[19] One attempt to compare the quality by means of performance on the registered nurse examinations in New York State as of July 1, 1968, is shown in Table 3–3.

A cursory comparison of the scores achieved by the associate degree (AD), the baccalaureate degree (DE), and the diploma (DI) programs shows:

1. The *highest* ranges are achieved by the baccalaureate degree nurses.
2. The *lowest* ranges of scores are shared by the diploma and associate degree graduates alike.
3. The diploma nurses achieve *higher* ranges of scores in all areas than do the associate degree nurses.
4. The average scores for the diploma students are *higher* in all areas than the average scores achieved by the associate degree nurses.
5. The *overall range* of scores achieved by the diploma nurse are *similar* to the baccalaureate degree nurse.

Comparisons based on these scores are tempered by the following limitations: Without knowing the standard deviation or

---

19. For convincing arguments for both sides of the controversy see Anne Kibrick, "Why Collegiate Programs for Nurses?," *New England Journal of Medicine* 278, no. 14 (April 4, 1968):765–72; Thomas Hale, "Cliches of Nursing Education," *New England Journal of Medicine* 278, no. 16 (April 18, 1968): 879–86.

Table 3–3. Range of Individual School Means, and Means of All Programs, by Type of Program on the Registered Professional Nursing Examinations in New York State, July 1, 1968[20]

Type	Level	Low	Mean	High
Medical	AD	397	447	533
	DE	447	537	621
	DI	394	516	606
Surgical	AD	391	450	545
	DE	416	516	588
	DI	324	504	569
Obstetric	AD	384	451	527
	DE	454	525	628
	DI	399	503	563
Pediatric	AD	370	443	519
	DE	449	533	638
	DI	377	514	608
Psychiatric	AD	421	474	530
	DE	460	569	645
	DI	392	507	595

Standard score 0   300   400   500   600   700   800

AD = Associate Degree. Two years.   DE = Degree (Baccalaureate). Four years.
DI = Diploma (Hospital Training). Three years.

numbers of schools in each of the three educational levels of programs, the significance of the differences among them cannot be measured statistically. A written examination is only one sample of

20. *An Abstract for Action*, p. 108.

performance; the scores are for New York State only; and the examination is written by the National League for Nursing, whose accreditation process has done much to enhance baccalaureate education. Hence, the examinations may be geared for baccalaureate students. However, one may conclude that the diploma graduates are closer in test achievement to the baccalaureate degree nurses than are the associate degree students who fall considerably short of either the diploma or baccalaureate performance.

As of 1972 there were 80,000 active baccalaureate nurses and nearly 580,000 diploma nurses.[21] By dint of numbers alone, diploma nurses are and will remain the majority group for many years to come. *Might nursing leadership do better to reconsider pursuit of higher education and pursue instead greater clinical expertise at all levels irrespective of educational preparation?*

Although its intention was to upgrade the profession, the ANA position paper has set one group in nursing against another—the diploma nurses against the baccalaureate nurses. Unfortunately, this house divided not only weakens nursing internally, but seriously compromises its clout in encounters with other professions. The results of the demise of hospital schools and the proliferation of the associate degree programs should be critically examined.

THE AMA–ANA CONFLICT

Although many doctors and nurses work well together at the patient's bedside, there is a recent history of friction between the nursing and medical organizations. Unfortunately this friction greatly impedes the ability of organized nursing and medicine to plan together toward the realization of improved patient care.

As mentioned earlier, the nurse was invited by the AMA in late 1969 to play an expanded role as an assistant. However, the AMA's overtures to nursing at that time were met with such rebuff that medicine then turned to the non-nurse physician's assistant. The effect of the physician's assistant movement on the ANA–AMA relationship is a fascinating process worth treating in greater detail.

The AMA Plan to Make Nurses into Physician's Assistants

The conflict between medicine and nursing erupted in February of 1970 when Dr. Ernest Howard, then AMA executive director, announced an AMA plan to make 100,000 nurses into

---

21. See Table 3–1, p. 25.

physician's assistants.[22] Specifically, doctors were urged to upgrade the professional skills of their office nurses by means of personal preceptorships. Under the physician's supervision the nurse would have direct patient responsibility, including house calls. The physician would bill for the nurse's services on his letterhead on a fee for service basis. Curiously, in voting for the new plan to expand the role of office nurses, the AMA board of trustees acted without prior consultation with organized nursing or even with their own AMA leaders who had special responsibilities pertaining to nursing. Nor was attention paid to the health insurers who would be asked to reimburse the fee for service billings to the nurse's account.

Nursing's Rebuttal

The response to the AMA plan by the then ANA president, Dorothy Cornelius, was immediate and wrathful: "The ANA board of directors deplores this kind of unilateral decision made by the AMA, since it is not the prerogative of the AMA to speak for any other profession. We strongly object to this action—that the AMA should attempt to meet the physician shortage by compounding the shortage of nurses."

NLN president Gwendoline MacDonald also was quick to deplore the AMA's unilateral action in delineating a new role for nurses. Among her points were that:

1. neither the NLN nor the ANA had been consulted on the proposal;
2. in spite of the innovation in expanded use of health personnel, it is unreasonable to rob one profession already depleted to meet the needs of another;
3. interdisciplinary cooperation and collaboration are necessary if common problems between medicine and nursing are to be solved.

Narrowing the Breach

One month later, on March 13, 1970, Dorothy Mereness, Dean of Nursing at the University of Pennsylvania, spanned the breach with her mediating address to the Council of Baccalaureate and Higher Degree Programs in Nursing of the NLN in Kansas City, Missouri. Her statement provided an unofficial nursing position until official statements of position could be crystallized. Noting the large

---

22. "AMA Unveils Surprise Plan to Convert R.N. Into Medic," *American Journal of Nursing* 70, no. 4 (April 1970):691–93; "AMA Urges Major New Role for Nurses," *American Medical News* (February 9, 1970).

numbers of registered nurses who choose not to practice because of "inadequate definitions of the nurse's roles in the organization, poor communication and coordination, and unreasonable work pressures," she made a plea to nursing leaders to assume a guiding role in conjunction with the AMA in the development of the nurse as a physician's associate. While agreeing in principle with Miss Cornelius, Miss Mereness expressed distress that

> the professional nursing organization had not already developed a position on this issue (the nurse as a physician's assistant) before the AMA issued its statement. During the last two years there have been many developments in relation to the physician's assistant about which the ANA was aware. It appears that this position of the AMA could become one of the most significant developments in modern nursing *without organized nursing having taken a position.*

She disagreed with her colleagues in baccalaureate nursing education who rejected the physician's assistant concept. "In spite of the misgivings of their colleagues, many graduate nurses will most certainly be interested in relating themselves to a physician and accepting whatever extra training he may deem necessary . . ." She had no quarrel with the concept of the nurse as an "associate" functioning in a collaborative role with a physician. "The introduction by the AMA of the nurse as the physician's assistant is probably the first of many dramatic changes to come."

In her final remarks she warned,

> The physician's assistant could be one opportunity for nurses to accept responsibilities beyond those usually expected of the well-prepared professional nurse. If members of organized nursing continue to view with alarm this development and others that are bound to come, they may be relegated to the role of observer and lose an opportunity to shape the destiny of the profession which they have served so steadfastly.

AMA–ANA Dialogue Begins—
The National Joint Practice Commission

A mere ten days after Mereness' speech, a top echelon meeting of the ANA and AMA was held at the ANA headquarters in New York City, and an ANA–NLN–AMA ad hoc committee formed to establish new channels of communication to discuss "congruent roles." In August 1971, this group agreed to proceed with the national and state joint practice commissions between medicine and nursing as recommended by the Lysaught report to "discuss and make recommendations concerning the congruent roles[23] of the physician and the nurse in providing quality health care, *with particular attention to the rise of the nurse master clinician; the introduction of the physician's assistant; the increased activity of other professions in areas long assumed to be the concern solely of the physician and/or the nurse*" (emphasis added).[24]

In January 1972, the ANA–AMA Joint Practice Commission,[25] made up of sixteen members, eight from each profession, was convened in St. Louis. Their goal is to establish optimum working relationships between medicine and nursing to assure the best care of patients.

Because the National Joint Practice Commission has been explicitly charged by the National Commission for the Study of Nursing and Nursing Education to give particular attention to the introduction of the physician's assistant, we think that limiting the composition at the outset to organized medicine and nursing may hamper its effectiveness. Why not have representatives of hospital administration, other health professions *including physician's assistants*, the law, business, and the public involved at the outset rather than "as early as progress in these joint discussions indicates"? Decisions by the AMA and the ANA will have hardened and a major opportunity to build a bridge between the physician's assistant and the nurse may be lost.

LYSAUGHT COMMISSION BROCHURE, "NURSE CLINICIAN AND PHYSICIAN'S ASSISTANT"

A supplementary brochure entitled "Nurse Clinician and Physician's Assistant: The Relationship Between Two Emerging Practitioner

---

23. In the past, agreements reached at the state level through joint committees generally have been limited to procedural questions [Can a nurse start intravenous fluids?], and not fundamental policy questions such as congruent roles.

24. *An Abstract For Action* p. 89.

25. Members of the original National Joint Practice Commission were: Genrose Alfano, M.S., R.N., Bronx, New York; Patricia Devine, M.S., R.N., Parsons, Kansas, Thomas F. Dillon, M.D., New York, New York; A. Alan Fischer, M.D., Indianapolis; Robert A. Hoekelman, M.D., Rochester, New York; Marilyn J. Howe, M.S., R.N., Cleveland; Joseph W. Marshall, M.D., Twin Falls, Idaho; Nancy Melvin, M.A., R.N., Phoenix, Arizona; William H. Muller, M.D., Charlottesville, Virginia; Robert A. Murray, M.D., Temple, Texas; Otto C. Page, M.D., Portland, Oregon; Anna Bower Sherlock, M.S., R.N., Tucson, Arizona; Shirley Smoyak, Ph.D., R.N., New Brunswick, New Jersey; Virginia Stone, Ph.D., R.N., Durham, North Carolina; Barbara Taylor, M.S., R.N., Boston; James W. Walker, M.D., Jacksonville, Florida. (Note that every nurse representative has a graduate degree.)

Concepts," was prepared by Dr. Lysaught. After a candid and articulate summary of the state of the art of nursing and the recognition that major changes are required, the brochure noted that

> two companion answers have been swelling simultaneously. One answer hinges on the presence of the existing body of American nurses, large in number, already trained in many of the areas that are commonly considered to be paramount to the new practice. A second, *competing*, answer hinges on the development of a new category of personnel, separately named, separately trained[26] (emphasis added).

We regard nursing and the PA as complementary, *not* competing, professions.

After assuming that the relationship between the commission recommendations and the rising interest in the physician's assistant is close and direct, the brochure warned:

> If the physician's assistant becomes, in fact, a foreclosure on the development of increased enhanced role functioning in nursing, then we think we are making a very serious mistake in terms of the long-run needs of the country. And we would hazard to suggest that it will be a serious mistake for the profession of medicine as well as nursing and the health system generally.[27]

After talk about "foreclosure," the brochure noted that nurses have "historically been a physician's first assistant since 1900." It recognized that the major need to encourage nurses to stay within the profession was job enlargement, but failed to consider the root question underlying such enlargement, namely that of dependence/independence.

The brochure continued:

> "Now it may be that our concerns over the physician's assistants are entirely groundless. That is, the new occupation may not function to stifle the natural development of the nursing role and the career perspective of that profession."[28]

The brochure gave no basis for their concerns.

The brochure continued:

> "Let us emphasize in this regard that we do not anticipate that such commissions would necessarily reject the concept of the physician's

---

26. "Nurse Clinician and Physician's Assistant" (see pp. 65–76).
27. Ibid., p. 73.
28. Ibid., p. 74.

assistants." Finally, the brochure asked that "we wait—and we use that term emphatically—for concerted proposals from the Joint Practice Commissions for the future development of congruent roles and professional responsibilities. . . ."[29]

We suspect that the Joint Practice Commission, using this approach, will still be in the station trying to decide whether to accept or reject the concept when the physician's assistant train goes by. We wish the Commission had shared Dorothy Mereness' sense of urgency about the influence of the physician's assistant and nursing, one upon the other, and the need to get on immediately with the necessary collaboration.

One Step Forward

The strained relations between nursing and medicine in 1970 were compounded further by the American Academy of Pediatrics which presented unilaterally developed guidelines for the expanded training of nursing personnel to the ANA's Division of Maternal and Child Health Nursing for their endorsement. The requested endorsement was refused by the ANA pending input by organized nursing. Subsequent collaboration between the ANA and the AAP resulted in the January 1971 joint guidelines on short term continuing education programs for pediatric nurse associates.[30] This document stands to date as one of the more substantial constructive collaborations between a medical specialty and nursing—a model for future coaction between the various medical and nursing specialties.

One Step Backward

Just as time seemed to be working its healing powers, deep wounds between medicine and nursing were reopened with the unsuccessful attempt of the New York State Nurses Association to sponsor an amendment of the state's Nursing Practice Act to define and specify the independence of the nursing function. Passed by both houses of the state legislature, the bill was vetoed on July 6, 1971 by Governor Rockefeller on advice of the New York State Medical Society and the Hospital Association of New York State. The NYSNA responded immediately by letter of July 13 to the governor's veto, giving vent to their dismay and anger, calling Rockefeller's action and thinking "illogical," "shocking," "appalling,"

---

29. Ibid., p. 75.
30. ANA Division on Maternal and Child Health Nursing Practice and the American Academy of Pediatrics, "Guidelines on Short-Term Continuing Education Programs for Pediatric Nurse Associates" (January 1971).

"offensive," "lacking understanding or knowledge," "contradictory," "schizophrenic," "scandalous," "embarrassing," and "frightening." In almost any other state this incident could be dismissed as a local brawl having little or no consequence for the professions at large. However, given the fact that New York City housed the official power center, the ANA, as well as a traditional locus of power in nursing education, Teachers College of Columbia University, these renewed hostilities between nursing and medicine lent themselves to maximum visibility. The bill was reintroduced in March 1972 and passed. The legislation is discussed in detail in the next chapter.

ANA Looks Ahead
On the one side, the AMA's position with regard to nursing has developed unilaterally, with communication between the AMA and ANA being strained. The AMA has insisted upon expressing its opinions on the subject of nursing despite the ANA's challenge to their right to do so. Unfortunately, some of the language of the AMA has stressed the nurse's services to the physician rather than to the patient. On the other side has been *organized* nursing's concern with preservation of power and pride, which has blinded it to the merits in new opportunities proposed by the AMA.

When the physician's assistant was created in 1965, nursing education had already begun to concern itself with making a greater impact on service. This concern was reiterated in the Lysaught commission's 1970 statement "a first priority is the re-establishment of practice as the first and proper end of nursing. . . . In short, it is absolutely imperative that we redirect the reinforcement schema in nursing from rewarding non-practice activities to rewarding those actions most closely related to the intrinsic satisfactions that induce persons into the profession initially."[31]

In this connection, the physician's assistant has served as an issue around which nursing has begun to move toward a rapprochement with organized medicine. The progress is typified by the May 1972 ANA convention clinical sessions which featured RN–MD teamwork. "Sharper focus is placed on the interdisciplinary approach to patient care demonstrated by a colleague relationship between nurse and physician."[32]

The fractious relationship between nursing and medicine over the past year appears to be mellowing. This is encouraging

---

31. "Nurse Clinician and Physician's Assistant."
32. "RN–MD Teamwork Feature of 1972 Clinical Sessions," *The American Nurse* 4, no. 1 (February 1972):1.

indeed and is to be applauded. It augurs a brighter future for health care delivery of which the physician's assistant will be a part.

As for the lessons from nursing, the PA movement should beware of being similarly co-opted by the status afforded education and the drive to independent professionalization.

Resource Document

Excerpts from "Educational Preparation for Nurse Practitioners and Assistants to Nurses"*

... ASSUMPTIONS

The premises or assumptions underlying the development of the position are:

Nursing is a helping profession and, as such, provides services which contribute to the health and well-being of people.

Nursing is of vital consequence to the individual receiving services; it fills needs which cannot be met by the person, by the family, or by other persons in the community.

The demand for services of nurses will continue to increase.

The professional practitioner is responsible for the nature and quality of all nursing care patients receive.

The services of professional practitioners of nursing will continue to be supplemented and complemented by the services of nurse practitioners[1] who will be licensed.

---

*A position paper prepared by the American Nurses' Association, December 1965.

1. The specific meanings of certain terms used in this paper are:
Nurse practitioner: any person prepared and authorized by law to practice nursing and, therefore, deemed competent to render safe nursing care.

Nursing service: the system through the services of nurse practitioners and their assistants are made available to those in need.

Health facilities: a specially designed place where people receive health instruction and care.

Health service occupations: defined by the U.S. Office of Education as those occupations that render supportive services to the health professions.

Preservice preparation: an organized program of instruction received prior to employment.

Inservice education: an organized program of instruction during employment.

Education for those in the health professions must increase in depth and breadth as scientific knowledge expands.

The health care of the public, in the amount and to the extent needed and demanded, requires the services of large numbers of health occupation workers, in addition to those licensed as nurses, to function as assistants to nurses. These workers are presently designated: nurses' aides, orderlies, assistants. attendants, etc.

The professional association must concern itself with the nature of nursing practice, the means for improving nursing practice, the education necessary for such practice, and the standards for membership in the professional association.

POSITION

Education for those who work in nursing should take place in institutions of learning within the general system of education.

Nursing practice has become complex and will continue to become even more so. The conditions of nursing, as that of any other professional service, are determined by the structure of society and its prevailing values.

To point out that the practice of nursing has changed in the last 20 years is to point out the obvious. Major theoretical formulations, scientific discoveries, technological innovations, and the development of radical new treatments in recent years have produced marked changes in health practices. The knowledge needed by the nurse practitioner today differs greatly from that needed 20 or even 10 years ago. She is now being required to master a complex, growing body of knowledge and to make critical, independent judgments about patients and their care.

It is recognition of this need for mastery of a complex body of knowledge, and the continuing need to learn and improve practice, that has led the association to believe that:

the education for all those who are licensed to practice nursing should take place in institutions of higher education.

Professional Nursing Practice

The essential components of professional nursing are care, cure, and coordination. The care aspect is more than "to take care of," it is "caring for" and "caring about" as well. It is dealing with human beings under stress, frequently over long periods of time. It is providing comfort and support in times of anxiety, loneliness, and helplessness. It is listening, evaluating, and intervening appropriately.

The promotion of health and healing is the cure aspect of professional nursing. It is assisting patients to understand their health problems and helping them to cope. It is the administration of medications and treatments. And it is the use of clinical nursing judgment in determining, on the basis of patients' reactions, whether the plan for care needs to be maintained or changed. It is knowing when and how to use existing and potential resources to help patients toward recovery and adjustment by mobilizing their own resources.

Professional nursing practice is this and more. It is sharing responsibility for the health and welfare of all those in the community and participating in programs designed to prevent illness and maintain health. It is coordinating and synchronizing medical and other professional and technical services as these affect patients. It is supervising, teaching, and directing all those who give nursing care.

Professional nursing practice is constant evaluation of the practice itself. It provides an opportunity for increasing self-awareness and personal and professional fulfillment. It is asking questions and seeking answers—the research that adds to the body of theoretical knowledge. It is using this knowledge, as well as other research findings, to improve services to patients and service programs to people. It is collaborating with those in other disciplines in research, in planning, and in implementing care. Further, it is transmitting the ever-expanding body of knowledge in nursing to those within the profession and outside of it.

Such practice requires knowledge and skill of high order, theory-oriented rather than technique-oriented. It requires education which can only be obtained through a rigorous course of study in colleges and universities. Therefore,

minimum preparation for beginning professional nursing practice at the present time should be baccalaureate degree education in nursing.

Yet it is obvious that all of the nursing needs of people cannot be met by the professional nurse practitioner alone. It is recognized that supporting personnel with considerable understanding of theory and a high degree of technical skill in the application of principles are needed to augment the efforts of the professional practitioner of nursing. This is due, in part, to a continuing trend toward specialization in all fields of endeavor and particularly in medical care. New knowledge and new machines almost daily render obsolete what has been learned in the past. The professional nurse practitioner alone cannot master all the measures necessary for the care of patients, nor all of the technology associated with cure. The association, therefore, takes the view that the technical aspects of nursing care and cure will assume even greater importance in the future. Nursing is not alone in this respect: science, engineering, architecture, business, and medicine have all recognized the important contribution which can be made by the technician.

Technical Nursing Practice

Technical nursing practice is carrying out nursing measures as well as medically delegated techniques with a high degree of skill, using principles from an ever-expanding body of science. It is understanding the physics of machines as well as the physiologic reactions of patients. It is using all treatment modalities with knowledge and precision.

Technical nursing practice is evaluating patients' immediate physical and emotional reactions to therapy and taking measures to alleviate distress. It is knowing when to act and when to seek more expert guidance.

Technical nursing practice involves working with professional nurse practitioners and others in planning the day to day care of patients. It is supervising other workers in the technical aspects of care.

Technical nursing practice is unlimited in depth but limited in scope. Its complexity and extent are tremendous. It must be rendered, under the direction of professional nurse practitioners, by persons who are selected with care and educated within the system of higher education; only thus can the safety of patients be assured. Education for this practice requires attention to scientific laws and principles with emphasis on skill. It is education which is technically-oriented and scientifically-founded, but not primarily concerned with evolving theory.

In many fields technical education long has been accepted as the responsibility of higher education—both junior and senior colleges. The non-degree-granting technical institute slowly is disappearing from the American scene. The movement of all types of education beyond high school into colleges and universities, and the growth and effectiveness of associate degree programs in nursing, are of significance to the nursing profession.

The issue—how the technical worker can achieve the status and prestige needed to perform a proper and vital role—is not an issue for nursing alone, but one which concerns the whole of society. The number of technical occupations is increasing rapidly; the ratio of technicals to professionals becomes larger as knowledge increases and society focuses more on production and distribution. Nursing can wait for the changes in society to alter attitudes and to spur an attack on this issue, or nursing can take the initiative. Therefore,

minimum preparation for beginning technical nursing practice at the present time should be associate degree education in nursing.

In addition to the services of nurse practitioners, people in need of health services require the services of health occupation workers who can function as assistants to nurses. These workers— nurses' aides, orderlies, nursing assistants, and others with on the job training—have long been employed by nursing services to perform delegated tasks in the care of the sick in the hospital. Such workers free the nurse practitioner to concentrate on those functions which she alone is prepared to assume. Because health services today are provided in homes as well as in a variety of organized health facilities, and because all health professions are utilizing the services of these auxiliary workers, hospital training courses conducted by nurses no longer are adequate or appropriate for training this group of workers. The functions of workers assisting in the health fields are sufficiently general in nature to be appropriate to many of the health and helping professions. Therefore,

education for assistants in the health service occupations should be short, intensive preservice programs in vocational education institutions rather than on the job training programs.

Most of this preservice preparation must be done by vocational educators who may not necessarily be nurses; if they are nurses, they should meet the qualifications for teaching set by vocational education.

In addition to general preservice preparation, workers assigned to nursing services should be given inservice orientation and on the job training to perform specific tasks delegated by nurses. This rule, that on the job orientation and continuing inservice education be followed through by the service to which the worker is assigned, should apply not only to nursing services but also to other health services in which these workers will assist.

The current role of government in financing programs to train workers for the health fields requires the nursing profession to enunciate standards for the education of all who share the activities of nursing. It should not, however, require that nursing assume responsibility for the standards and preparation of those who function as assistants to personnel in other health professions. . . .

IMPLICATIONS

It is obvious that the association's first position on education for nursing has implications for present-day nursing education, nursing practice, nursing service, and the training of auxiliary workers.

Responsibility for the education of nurses historically has been carried by hospitals, and the graduates of hospital-based diploma programs comprise approximately 78 percent of nurses now in practice. However, economic pressures on the hospital, and other developments in society, are increasing the movement of nursing education programs into the colleges and universities, the loci of education for all other professions.

In the light of what can be seen at present, it is reasonable to expect that many diploma schools of nursing will participate with colleges and universities in planning for the development of baccalaureate programs; others will participate with junior colleges in planning for the development of associate degree programs. Both senior and junior college programs will need hospitals and other health resources in the community as laboratories.

Colleges and universities not now offering programs in nursing, but having the resources to do so, must be made aware of their responsibility to society to provide education for practitioners in nursing.

Colleges and universities now offering programs in nursing must be made aware of their responsibility to expand facilities and faculties to accommodate the expected increased numbers of applicants. Such expansion, however, can only take place if increased numbers of master clinical practitioners are prepared to assume faculty positions.

Colleges and universities must also determine the distinctions between education which prepares technical nurse practitioners and that which prepares professional nurse practitioners so that applicants for nursing programs enter those programs for which they best qualify.

In addition, colleges and universities must carry on programs for continuing education, advanced study, and research in nursing in order to provide practitioners with up to date knowledge and skill and advanced theory, and add to the fund of knowledge in nursing.

Practical nursing has become a major occupational group in a few short years. Practical nurses have made a significant contribution to the care of patients in the absence of adequate numbers of registered nurses. Practical nurses also, more often than not, are expected to carry job responsibilities beyond those for which they are educated. The job demands made on them are those which more nearly approach those for which the registered nurse is educated. Increasingly, more complex activities have been delegated to practical nurses and, increasingly, their preservice preparation has become more complex, requiring a higher level of ability. In some regions, preparation for practical nursing now takes 18 months, and there have been proposals for programs of two years in length, some in junior colleges. The association, therefore, proposes that the nursing profession acknowledge these changes and systematically work to facilitate the replacement of programs for practical nursing with programs for beginning technical nursing practice in junior and community colleges.

CONCLUSION

The ultimate aim of nursing education and nursing service is the improvement of nursing care. The primary aim of each is different.

The primary aim of nursing education is to provide an environment in which the nursing student can develop self-discipline, intellectual curiosity, and the ability to think clearly, and acquire the knowledge necessary for practice. Nursing education reaches its utlimate aim when recent advances in knowledge and findings from nursing research are incorporated into the program of study in nursing.

The primary aim of nursing service is to provide nursing care of the type needed, and in the amount required, to those in need of nursing care. Nursing service reaches its ultimate aim when it provides a climate where questions about practice can be raised and answers sought, where nursing staffs continue to develop and learn, and where nurses work collaboratively with persons in other disciplines to provide improved services to patients.

These aims—educating nurses and providing patients with care—can only be carried out when nurses in education and in service recognize their interdependence and actively collaborate to achieve the ultimate aim of both—improved nursing care. . . .

"Nurse Clinician and Physician's Assistant: The Relationship between Two Emerging Practitioner Concepts"* *(Lysaught Brochure)*

In June of 1970, the National Commission for the Study of Nursing and Nursing Education announced the results and recommendations of a three year investigation of this profession and its relationship to health care in the United States. The impetus for this study can be traced directly to the 1963 report of the surgeon general's Consultant Group on Nursing which recommended in its final document, *Toward Quality in Nursing*, that there should be an independent examination of nursing with special emphasis on the responsibilities and skills required for high quality patient care.

In April of 1966, W. Allen Wallis, chancellor of the University of Rochester, agreed to head such a study if adequate financing could be arranged. The Avalon Foundation, The Kellogg Foundation, and individual benefactors collaborated in the support of the project, and it was officially begun in the fall of 1967 with the appointment of a study staff. The twelve members of the commission[1] met at

---

*Prepared by the National Commission for the Study of Nursing and Nursing Education for the Federation of State Medical Boards of the United States, February 12, 1971.

1. The original commission included: Ray Everett Brown, Executive Vice President, Northwestern University Medical Center; Dr. Lowell T. Coggeshall, former Vice President, University of Chicago; Margaret B. Dolan, Head, Department of Public Health Nursing, School of Public Health, University of North Carolina; Marion B. Folsom, former Secretary of Health, Education and Welfare; Walter E. Hoadley, Executive Vice President, Bank of America National Trust and Savings Association; Dr. Eleanor Lambertsen, Dean, School of Nursing, Cornell University; Dr. Herbert E. Longenecker, President, Tulane University; Mary Jane McCarthy, Director, Nursing Service, Veterans Administration; Leonard F. McCollum, Chairman of the Board, Continental Oil Company; Dr. Robert K. Merton, Giddings Professor of Sociology, Columbia University; Dr. Ralph W. Tyler, former Director, Center for Advanced Study in Behavioral Sciences, Stanford University; W. Allen Wallis, President, University of Rochester.

periodic intervals over the course of the next two and one-half years, and unanimously agreed on the culminating statement, *An Abstract for Action,*[2] which spoke to the problems of our health system, the pivotal role of nursing in the delivery of care, and the changes that are required in order to make the profession a full contributor to the solution of our difficulties.

In the months since the appearance of the final report, a number of actions have taken place. First, the Kellogg Foundation has enthusiastically agreed to fund an implementation phase to facilitate the adoption of the changes recommended. This has been followed by endorsement of the report by the American Nurses' Association, the National League for Nursing, and the Committee on Nursing of the American Medical Association; an ad hoc committee named by the American Hospital Association to study the report has reacted favorably to the central thrust of the recommendations and their statement has been accepted for the association on the recommendation of their general council. The Conference of Catholic Schools of Nursing, the New England Board of Higher Education, the Council of Deans and Directors of Southern Regional Education Board's Collegiate Nursing Programs, and the National Federation of Leagues of Practical Nursing are among other professional bodies that have given their support to the commission report.

These propitious events are not unexpected, because the study itself involved literally hundreds of individuals and groups, not only from nursing, but from medicine, health administration, allied health, education, health insurers, and that increasingly vocal body known as consumers—in some other contexts known as patients.

It was the openness and the objectivity of the approaches, further detailed in *An Abstract for Action, Volume II,*[3] that played a vital role in the planning for implementation. Believing both that definite action was required, and that the composition of the commission should be expanded to facilitate movement, Dr. Leroy E. Burney, then Vice President for Health Affairs at Temple University, and now President of the Milbank Memorial Fund, agreed to accept the presidency of the commission for the implementation phase. He was joined by the following new members: Dorothy A. Cornelius, Ohio Nurses' Association; Dr. Joseph Hamburg, The University of Kentucky; Dr. James Haughton, Cook County Hospitals Governing

---

2. National Commission for the Study of Nursing and Nursing Education, *An Abstract for Action* (New York: McGraw–Hill, 1970).

3. National Commission for the Study of Nursing and Nursing Education, *An Abstract for Action, Volume II, Appendices* (New York: McGraw–Hill, 1971).

Commission; Dr. C. A. Hoffman, AMA Board of Trustees; Dr. William N. Hubbard, Jr., The Upjohn Company; Boisfeuillet Jones, Emily and Ernest Woodruff Foundation; Mrs. Lois Turner Jones, The Playhouse Academy; Dr. Anne Kibrick, Boston College Department of Nursing; Stuart J. Marylander, Cedars-Sinai Medical Center; Charles S. Paxson, Jr., Hahnemann Medical College and Hospital; Dr. John D. Porterfield, Joint Commission on Accreditation of Hospitals; Mrs. Barbara Resnik, University of California School of Medicine; and Dr. Harold B. Wise, Martin Luther King Health Center.

Six of the original members of the commission continued on the board; Mrs. Margaret B. Dolan; Marion B. Folsom; Dr. Eleanor Lambertsen; Mary Jane McCarthy; Leonard F. McCollum; and Dr. Ralph W. Tyler. All other former commissioners have agreed to continue service on a national advisory council and to remain associated with the general activities of implementation.

This brief background to the commission and its work will underline the fact that experienced and outstanding individuals from all the health-related fields have joined forces to effect fundamental changes in the practice and educational patterns of the nursing profession.

THE EMERGENCE OF THE PHYSICIAN'S ASSISTANT CONCEPT

The growth of interest in, and actual development of preparatory programs for, physician's assistants has closely paralleled the time line of our nursing investigation. It can be reasonably inferred that the underlying problems which caused national concern for the future of nursing also sparked the interest in emerging health occupations. Among the trends that have evoked particular pleas for change are these:

1. *The Rising Need for Care.* A steadily expanding population coupled with increased concern for the inclusion of previously neglected societal segments has brought our entire health care system to the breaking point under sheer "people pressure." Even with a reduction in the birth rate, the increased base will provide vast numbers of new infants who require proportionately more than average amounts of health care. Additionally, the very success of our health care system has increased life expectancy and, concomitantly, the numbers of our geriatric and domiciliary patients beyond all past experience. Again, these individuals require more than average amounts of care. To meet these

demands, it requires little prescience to recognize that we need more hands. It may, however, be important for us to deliberate on what those hands are required to do and how skilled they must be in order to minister to the patients' needs.

2. *The Changed Economics of Health.* Accompanying the rise in demand for care is a fundamental change in the economic structure of our health system. Most analysts agree that, by 1975, 100 percent of our population will be covered (for all practical purposes) by some combination of public and private insurance systems. The short and middle range effects of such a development are bound to increase demands—now fortified with the assurance of prepayment—on an already creaking health system. Add to this the fact that more Americans, encouraged by their insurance for basic care, are spending increasing proportions of their discretionary income on cosmetic or marginal care, and we have the specter of demand almost choking the supply of health care through our present schema.

3. *Growing Interdependence of Care.* If there were no "outside" demands for greater care and greater numbers of care providers, the miracles of medical science would have required a basic re-examination of our staffing and role practices anyway. As Garfield[4] rather clearly documents, we have moved from a relatively simple doctor-patient relationship (circa 1900) that embodied most forms of treatment, to a highly complex, interdependent, and increasingly technological system of care. Transplant teams of 60 individuals, cardiac care units with disciplined groups of specialists administering highly technical procedures, new occupations, new disciplines, new equipment—and all interdependent in ways that were not imagined when we built most of our institutions and developed their staffing arrangements.

Little wonder, then, that both physician and layman join in a swelling cry for help. And little wonder that the concept of another care provider is advanced. A care provider who does not have all the skills of a physician; perhaps an individual who has some skills that the doctor does not develop or maintain. A care provider who can be educated more expeditiously, at less expense, and in more institutions than is the physician. Yet, overall, someone who is competent and humane in dispensing his much-needed services.

The basic question is not whether the physician needs help. He does. The basic question revolves around what kind of

4. Sidney R. Garfield, "The Delivery of Medical Care," *Scientific American* 222,4 (April 1970):15–23.

help—and by whom. And it is significant to all our concerns that two companion answers have been swelling simultaneously. One answer hinges on the presence of the existing body of American nurses, large in number, already trained in many of the areas that are commonly considered to be paramount to the new practice. A second, competing answer hinges on the development of a new category of personnel, separately named, separately trained. It is in this domain that the report of the national commission has particular relevance.

THE PARADOX OF NURSING

It is likely that the confusion of roles and planning begins with the very paradox of nursing itself. For one thing, the public and the health professions, even nursing itself, are conditioned to the existence of a nursing shortage. And these many individuals could scarcely be criticized for neglecting nursing in the consideration of changing roles in health care if they perceive the profession as being unable to fulfill its own manpower requirements.

As Yett and the other dissenters to the Nurse Training Act report maintain, however, there is a serious question about the shortage of nurses.[5] It has been reasonably estimated that we produce enough nurse graduates each year to provide an adequate supply of practitioners. Our problem comes first in the distinction between "need" and real economic demand. If Yett is correct, there may be a need for more nurses, but that need is not translated into real demand—otherwise defined perhaps as dollars—which can effectively induce the nurse into continued exercise of skills and training.

Not only has the nursing profession increased its overall numbers, but the ratio of nurses to population has increased steadily. In fact, in the period 1950 to 1968, nursing increased from 249 practitioners per 100,000 population to 338—at a time when medicine was making valiant efforts to increase the supply of physicians and was able to increase the ratio of doctors from 141 to only 150 per 100,000.

Any enthusiasm over this occurrence is rapidly chastened, however, when we examine the withdrawal rate from the nursing profession. While we have certainly increased the numbers and ratio of nurses in practice, we have suffered sobering losses from the potential numbers we might have attained. . . . One out of every four is totally inactive; another 25 percent is active only to the extent of maintaining licensure; of the remaining 50 percent almost one out of

---

5. Donald E. Yett, "The Nursing Shortage and the Nurse Training Act of 1964," *Industrial and Labor Relations Review* 29,1 (January 1966):200.

every three is a part time nurse. Of more than 1,300,000 graduate nurses, approximately 450,000 are employed full time. This figure, of course, includes nurse educators, administrators, supervisors, and all manner of practitioners.

Nor is the rate of inactivity the only disturbing evidence of trouble within the profession. Approximately one out of every three students who enter any kind of preparatory program in nursing drop out before completion of their program. Not only do nurses display a greater rate of withdrawal from their profession than any other group of women with similar education and training, but the average rate of turnover among staff nurses in American hospitals is over 70 percent while the rate of turnover among elementary and secondary teachers—also predominantly female and from the same socioeconomic backgrounds—is approximately 20 percent. Finally, there has been a slow but steady decline in the percentage of high school graduates selecting nursing as an occupational choice.[6]

As indicated by the brief comparisons to other "women's groups" it is inaccurate and misleading to explain these problems by the mere statement that nurses are women and that is that! At the risk of oversimplification, our three year analysis of these complex problems wholly corroborated the argument of Hoekelman who proposes, "By any of the criteria which define a shortage of personnel in any occupation, one cannot claim a shortage of registered nurses in this country."[7] *This does not mean, of course, that there is not a need for more practitioners.* It does emphasize that our past approaches to the problems and our assessment of solutions have been naive.

In terms of our present knowledge of industrial and social psychology, it is useful to view the continuation of career performance in terms of a concept of social behavior based on the presence or absence of rewards—in more precise psychological terms, reinforcement. This view, rather than accepting a shortage of personnel as a condition, sees it as a result. And, in terms of the available manpower pool in nursing, this seems a reasonable beginning.

Social psychology would approach the problem in terms like this: the social behavior of nursing is reinforced by a variety of benefits; if the sum total of these benefits is both truly rewarding, and relatively more rewarding than other alternative occupations,

---

6. See also The National Commission for the Study of Nursing and Nursing Education, "A Guide for Establishing Statewide Joint Practice Commissions," *pamphlet* (Rochester, N.Y.:1970).

7. Robert A. Hoekelman, "Florence's Fable," *Newsletter of the Ambulatory Pediatric Association* 5,2 (February 1970):23.

then we would expect to find an increased duration of individual activity in the career, reduced turnover, lowered rates of withdrawal, and other evidence of career satisfaction. On the other hand, if the sum total of real, and relative, benefits is inadequate, we would expect to find high withdrawal, high turnover, and frustration symptoms within the occupation and its career patterns. If this last statement is not a description of American nursing today, then we would not know how to put it into words.

In the light of such an analysis, nursing basically suffers from a lack of sufficiently rewarding conditions. The result is personnel shortage and serious morale problems—neither of which can be resolved until the basic conditions are overcome.

Social reinforcers may be viewed as being either extrinsic or intrinsic to the basic needs of the individual. Extrinsic reinforcers, such as pay and benefits, can provide for the basic survival and security needs of the individual as suggested by Maslow.[8] Such a formulation suggests that until the basic needs of the individual for a living wage and reasonable economic security have been met, it is generally useless to appeal to other motives as a springboard to action. That there are evident economic concerns over nursing compensation is widely recognized. The emphasis of the nursing organizations on economic security, the increasing militancy of bargaining, the development of nursing unions, and the growth of the entire "fem lib" salary protest dramatically score the need to provide more reasonable levels—and prospects—of compensation. Parenthetically, however, we would state that economic problems are the most easily solved despite their complexity. Our genius for business in America, and the structure of our modified capitalist society, suggest that we are well geared to handling salary and compensation matters once we identify and really set out to tackle them.

Important as these extrinsic satisfactions are to the individual, Maslow emphasizes that there exists a hierarchy of needs and that each individual has a satiety level for each area of rewards. When this personal satisfaction point is reached, then we must begin to operate with different kinds of rewards. Herzberg[9] is even more emphatic in his consideration of motivational factors because he suggests that certain kinds of rewards are hygienic, merely preventing dissatisfaction, while another group of reinforcers actually produce job and career satisfaction.

---

8. Abraham Maslow, *Motivation and Personality* (New York: Harper and Brothers, 1954).

9. Frederick Herzberg, Bernard Mausner, and Barbara Snyderman. *The Motivation to Work* (New York: John Wiley and Sons, 1959).

The point to conjure with is whether there are indeed some intrinsic satisfiers in nursing that could not only provide a long range solution to its manpower problems, but contribute to the revitalization of our health care system. The answer may be so simple and direct as to be overlooked. If we examine the abundant evidence of Hughes[10] and others, we will recognize that the primary reason for entering nursing at all is expressed in the desire "to help people." This would suggest in pretty straightforward fashion that the individuals themselves identify as behavioral reinforcers those activities related to direct patient care functions and, very likely, the ability to increase systematically the quality of such personal activity.

If these are the most critical dimensions of intrinsic reinforcement, then we could not have developed a more diabolical approach to frustrating the individual nurse than the present utilization patterns we employ. Christman and Helinek[11] report after intensive study that registered nurses in hospital situations spend 50 to 75 percent of their time in nonnursing functions. Their results are confirmed by Duff and Hollingshead,[12] and by many other researchers. In fact, in the analyses we studied of nursing utilization, the RN spent less time in direct patient care than did the practical nurse, the orderly, other types of staff personnel, and the student nurse. We know the temptation is to say: "Well, that's the way they like it." Our reply is that the ones who stay may like it, but most nurses get out of that situation either entirely or through choosing alternative professional paths.

These alternative professional paths include the movement into nursing education and administration—the recognized positions of power and added compensation. If the frustrations do not drive the nurses away, then the skewed reinforcement system strongly tends to attract them out of practice. And yet, practice is the primary area of higher intrinsic satisfaction—unless the accumulated testimony of thousands of nurses is to be cast aside without consideration.

It is for these reasons that a first priority of the national commission, in terms of recommendations, is the reestablishment of practice as the first and proper end of nursing as a profession. For this purpose, we have recommended research into the basics of practice and the development of educational curricula in terms of

---

10. Everett Hughes et al. *Twenty Thousand Nurses Tell Their Story* (Philadelphia: J. B. Lippincott Company, 1958).
11. Luther P. Christman and R. C. Jelinek, "Old Patterns Waste Half the Nursing Hours," *Modern Hospital* 8,1 (January 1967):79.
12. R. S. Duff and A. B. Hollingshead. *Sickness and Society* (New York: Harper and Row, 1968).

clinical requirements based on those research findings. Perhaps the commission philosophy is best summed up in their statement that ". . . . nursing career patterns should be so organized that recognition, reward, and increased responsibility . . . are based on increasing depth of knowledge and demonstrated competence to perform in complex clinical situations." In short, it is absolutely imperative that we redirect the reinforcement schema in nursing from rewarding nonpractice activities to rewarding those actions most closely related to the intrinsic satisfactions that induce persons into the profession initially. And this is not suggested for the purpose of "making the nurses happy," but as a cold, hard design to ensure that our health care system remains viable.

RELATIONSHIP TO THE PHYSICIAN'S ASSISTANT

We assume by this point that the relationship between the commission recommendations and the rising interest in the physician's assistant is close and direct. If the physician's assistant becomes, in fact, a foreclosure on the development of increased, enhanced role functioning in nursing then we think we are making a very serious mistake in terms of the long run needs of the country. And we would hazard to suggest that it will be a serious mistake for the profession of medicine as well as nursing and the health system generally.

The chairman of the AMA Committee on Nursing, Dr. Charles Leedham, points out:

> The nurse is the logical individual to support the physician in the management and care of the patient. This support is broadened as nursing moves into the age of specialization. This thrust toward an expanded role supports the desire expressed by the nursing profession for more significant role responsibilities. An enhanced role for the nurse will enable the physician-nurse team to better meet the challenging demand for more adequate delivery of health care to the entire population.[13]

Proceeding on the simple facts that the nurse has historically been the physician's first assistant since 1900; that nursing represents the largest single body of prepared health practitioners in the country; and that nurses are forcefully expressing an interest in enhanced role practice in both episodic and distributive settings, it seems only rational to plan jointly before we once more recapitulate

13. Eileen M. Jacobi, "Officially Speaking . . . ," *RN Magazine* 33,10 (1970):57, 82–84.

the fatal cycle of setting up one more health occupation that must fight for its place in the sun by coopting the functions and techniques of its related functionaries.

It is strange indeed that we show so little willingness to learn from the experience of those whose professional study is the examination of organizational effectiveness. At the very time we in the health sector are emphasizing the development, nay proliferation, of more and more occupations of more and more limited scope, the people who have examined the scientific management model in business and industry (over a much longer period and under more controled conditions than we in the health professions) are rejecting such approaches for the opposite concept of job enlargement. And we know of no more apt way of describing both the natural desires of nursing and the requirement for developing the environment for intrinsic motivation than to label it as "job enlargement."

Now it may be that our concerns over the physician's assistant are entirely groundless. That is, the new occupation may not function to stifle the natural development of the nursing role and the career perspective of that profession. As a matter of fact, the variety of programs labeled as preparatory for the physician's assistant makes it difficult for us to analyze precisely what we mean by the term. But this brings us to the point that the public interest, the need for interdependence in professional role performance, and our own need to function effectively argue against another experience of "muddling through" the problem. To this end, the national commission has a proposal that we think is critical for all our sakes. The commission recommends that we begin to think and plan first, then act in accordance with consensual decisions. Specifically, we propose that:

> A National Joint Practice Commission, with state counterpart committees, be established between medicine and nursing to discuss and make recommendations concerning the congruent roles of the physician and the nurse in providing quality health care with particular attention to the rise of the nurse clinician; the introduction of the physician's assistant; the increased activity of other professions and skills in areas long assumed to be the concern solely of the physician and/or the nurse.

This specific proposal, central to the thrust of the report as a whole, has been endorsed by both the ANA Board of Directors and the AMA Board of Trustees and represents a viable alternative to the growth of occupations "like Topsy." A beginning has been made in implementation of this recommendation through the joint committee of the AMA–ANA–NLN, but more specific attention must be given to the congruent role concerns of the practitioners—and that should be the province of a newly appointed Joint Practice Commission. A beginning has already been made through joint agreement of the ANA Congress for Nursing Practice and the AMA Committee on Nursing. From their cooperation can come the foundation of the National Joint Practice Commission.

Through national and state counterpart committees we can begin to resolve the functional and jurisdictional problems that have beset us for too long—and hopefully prevent their proliferation and reoccurrence. Let us emphasize in this regard that we do not anticipate that such commissions would necessarily reject the concept of the physician's assistants. Rather, we would hope they could better clarify the roles of such a person, determine whether such an individual needs to be developed *ab initio* or can be drawn from established manpower pools, and outline the relationships of such a person to related role performers.

RELATED ADMINISTRATIVE MATTERS

While we wait—and we use that term emphatically—for concerted proposals from the joint practice commissions for the future development of congruent roles and professional responsibilities, the commission feels strongly that we should retain our current licensing regulations in nursing, that is, a single license attesting to minimal skills for safe beginning practice. The certification of advanced clinical practice, specialization, and other recognized level of professional competence should for now be left to professional—or interprofessional—boards. We recognize that the decisions which come from the joint practice commissions will have a decided impact on the health practice laws of the several states since it seems inevitable that nursing will assume both more responsibility and liability for individual practice in all kinds of settings. We have already had experience in more than half the states with the formulation of joint statements on practice which have affected either state practice acts or their specific interpretation. Likely, the emergent roles will require more fundamental reconstruction of governing legislation than can be accomplished by simple amendment or rulings.

This, however, we recognize as the forte of the state practice boards. And it is presumptuous of us to enlarge upon it. Suffice it to say that the state medical boards can be decisive in the development of new and congruent roles between the two oldest health professions—not for the purpose of barring the development of new occupations, but to ensure orderly, rational, and effective emergence of needed health practitioners in place of a proliferation of idiosyncratic role developments.

Resource Document

"The American Nurses' Association Views the Emerging Physician's Assistant"*

Demands for health care services are rising sharply. At the same time, manpower needs in industry and agriculture are decreasing, so that employment must be found for more people in the service fields. The search for means to meet the health care demands and the need for new areas of employment are creating pressures for new careers in the health field.

One of the most significant among the emerging occupations is the "physician's assistant." A variety of training programs are being developed to prepare individuals to assist the physician. *The term "physician's assistant" should not be applied to any of the nurse practitioners being prepared to function in an extension of the nursing role.* However, the term appropriately can be applied in the training and utilization of persons who under medical direction assist physicians by performing specific delegated medical activities. Some of these individuals are now organizing and seeking recognition as a distinct group of practitioners in health care.

The American Nurses' Association views all nurse practitioners as members of the nursing profession. ANA assumes responsibility for defining the scope of their practice, for determining standards and educational requirements, and for interpreting their ethical and legal relationships with physicians.

The practice of nursing is authorized by the nursing practice acts of the states. A joint practice commission composed of representatives of ANA and the American Medical Association has been established to consider the congruent roles of nurses and physicians. This development holds promise for more effective and efficient utilization of the two major health professions in future health care services.

---

*Prepared by the ANA Board of Directors, December 17, 1971.

Several types of assistants are being prepared and utilized to function under medical direction to extent physicians' services. None of these assistants are prepared to be substitutes for nurses, since nursing practice is more than performance of delegated medical nursing activities. Neither are these assistants acceptable substitutes for physicians. This development is of concern to the nursing profession. Physician's assistants working in a setting where nursing practice is an essential element of health care present problems that flow from the legal and ethical relationships between physicians and nurses. Therefore, nurses and physicians together must clarify the situation.

As yet there are no generally accepted guidelines for the preparation of all of these assistants. Further, there are as yet no universally accepted guidelines for the utilization of physician's assistants within the delivery system. Because of the vast differences in current programs, it is essential that efforts be made to bring about some uniformity of educational requirements.

As other groups have done in the past, physician's assistants are becoming organized in an effort to secure licensure, certification and other forms of recognition as a distinct health occupation. Until the functions of the physician's assistant are more clearly identified, and generally acceptable standards for training and practice are evident, licensure for their practice by the states should not be attempted.

The American Nurses' Association supports the call for a moratorium on the licensure of new categories of health workers until studies have been conducted to determine the need for licensure reform. Prior to such reform, it is imperative that the medical profession retain responsibility for delegation of medical acts to physician's assistants.

In licensing law, it first should be possible to define an independent area of practice which must be regulated in the interest of public health and safety. The definition of any health profession's practice should be stated in terms that are broad enough to permit flexibility in the utilization of assisting personnel within the bounds of safety for the client. The definition should also permit changes in practice consistent with desirable trends in health care practices.

Because the economic status of each group involved in health care is part of the economic environment of every other group, the American Nurses' Association has a stake in the economic status of the emerging physician's assistant. The ANA reemphasizes that in establishing salary systems, recognition must be given to the character of responsibilities carried, and to requirements for education, experience, and clinical expertise. In establishing the relationships between salaries of nurses and those of physician's assistants the differences in their responsibilities, preparation, and experience should be taken into account.

The development of new health workers has provided impetus for long overdue examination of the health care system including the responsibility of each health worker for providing service to the patient. The focus must become people, their health needs, and meeting these needs through high quality care and in the most efficient and economic manner feasible.

"Massachusetts Nurses Association Position Statement on the Physician's Assistant"*

Whereas, In spite of gallant efforts to alter the way in which nursing is able to function in our nonsystem of health care, progress has been slow in some areas and nonexistent in others. This disappointing situation is due, in part at least, to the fact that tinkering with one aspect of the system is not what is needed. Instead, this country requires a complete reorganization of the way in which health care is delivered; and

Whereas, As the largest of the health professions, and as one of our most precious resources, nursing must function at its best if we are to meet the demand for episodic and distributive care. . . . , nursing must be allowed—and required—to practice at its very highest capability. and thereby nursing accepts its inherent responsibilities for independent as well as collaborative functioning; and

Whereas, The redefinition of roles in medicine and nursing is ongoing; and

Whereas, There has been a proliferation of health workers and random development of educational programs, and varying degrees of educational prerequisites; and

Whereas, The practice settings of health workers differ; and

Whereas, There has been inconsistent supervision of health practices; and

Whereas, There has been a lack of statutory control of health practices; therefore,

Resolved, That we support the development of an orderly identification, through collaborative action of responsible profes-

---

*Released in March 1971.

sional groups, of essential health care professionals and other health workers to provide for the changing health needs of our society.

Resolved, That we support planning, implementation and evaluation of educational programs to ensure that other health workers are adequately prepared in mutual cooperation with all health care professionals to meet the health needs of society.

Resolved, That we strongly reinforce that the professional bodies of medicine and nursing are the major collaborators in, and that other health workers are resources who enhance, the delivery of primary health care.

Resolved, That we strongly urge that the sociolegal dimensions of the physician's assistant practices be clarified and clearly articulated in order to enable health groups to identify their interrelationships.

Resolved, That we recommend that employers and/or facilities accept their inferred responsibility to develop and implement standards and policies consistent with existing statutes regarding the practice of this health worker.

Resolved, That we recommend that all statutes and pending legislation related to the deliverers of health care be reviewed and/or developed with regard to prevailing roles and relationships of health professionals to allow for safe and congruent assimilation of new health care practices.

"New York State Nurses Association's Statement on the Physician's Associate and Specialist's Assistant"*

The emergence of two new categories of health workers in New York State, the physician's associate and specialist's assistant,[1] is unquestionably a tribute to the medical profession's concern and vision regarding the increasing demand for medical care services. This development documents clearly that profession's recognition of the deleterious consequences of the unavailability of such services to the people of this state. Further, it reflects the medical profession's commitment and determination to improve the present unsatisfactory situation.

The New York State Nurses Association has long supported the concept of a clearly identified assistant to the physician. The association wishes to reaffirm that support and to welcome these new members of the health care team. Obviously, implementation of these roles will not only enhance medical practice, but more importantly will provide for more effective utilization of the unique talents and services of nursing practitioners. Therefore, the association pledges every cooperation in the orderly and efficient integration of these workers into the health care delivery system. In order to augment such integration the association wishes to clarify its position on this development as it relates to the nursing profession.

The association's position is as follows:

1. *The role of the nursing practitioner is not synonymous with that of the physician's associate or the specialist's assistant.*

The association is compelled to emphasize this distinction in light

---

*Approved by the NYSNA Board of Directors, January 31, 1972.
1. Hereafter in this statement the term "physician's assistant" shall refer to the physician's associate and specialist's assistant.

of the persistent lack of understanding and recognition of the nature of nursing practice. Nursing practitioners, physicians, and physician's associates—indeed, all health care workers—must necessarily share common bodies of knowledge and overlapping areas of functional expertise. However, to assume "interchangeability" of roles is to deny the uniqueness of each, thus diminishing the capability for meeting society's complex health care needs.

2. *The physician's associate or specialist's assistant is not a substitute for the physician.*

The association recognizes the right of the medical profession to determine those medical acts which may be safely delegated to physician's assistants. Similarly, as an independent profession, nursing reserves the right to determine from whom it shall accept "delegation." Hence, nursing practitioners shall continue to execute those medical regimens prescribed only by a licensed or otherwise legally authorized physician or dentist.

In view of the original intent of the physician's assistant role, i.e., to increase the availability of medical care services to the public, the association questions the rationale for consideration of assigning the assistant to write medical orders. It would appear that such utilization unnecessarily limits the assistant's involvement in direct services to patients. However, if the medical profession deems it appropriate to assign to the physician's assistant the task of writing medical orders, then the association believes it appropriate for the physician's assistant to also carry out those orders.

3. *The salary schedules for physician's assistants should reflect not only health care costs in general and the particular skills and competencies required for these positions, but also equitable relationships with the salaries and fees of other health workers.*

In keeping with its long standing policy the association will continue to insure appropriate financial compensation for services rendered by nursing practitioners and maintain an appropriate relationship between nurses' salaries and fees and those of other members of the health care team. The association will scrutinize very carefully the impact of salary schedules of the physician's assistant on the recruitment and retention of other members of the health care team.

The New York State Nurses Association endorses the view of the American Nurses' Association relative to the physician's assistant.[2] This association also supports the American Nurses' Association's attempt to maintain dialogue on this matter with the American Medical Association and the American Hospital Association. Consistent with this, the New York State Nurses Association shall continue its effort toward comparable collaboration with the Medical Society of the State of New York, and the Hospital Association of New York State and those state governmental agencies charged with implementation of physician's assistant legislation.

2. American Nurses' Association, *The American Nurses Association Views the Emerging Physician's Assistant* (New York: The Association, December 1971).

Chapter Four

Where the Law Intervenes

THE MALPRACTICE MYTH

Concern has been expressed that the utilization of physician's assistants will increase malpractice risks. In light of the enormous number and size of malpractice verdicts being rendered today and our increasingly "suit-conscious" society, this concern is natural.

However, it is too early to know whether the use of physician's assistants will actually increase malpractice litigation. To our knowledge, no graduate of a university medical school physician's assistant program has been sued for malpractice. We will dispense quickly with the malpractice problem, which in our opinion will prove to be largely a myth, before analyzing the critical legal issues.

In our view, the utilization of well-trained physician's assistants who perform tasks within their capacity under appropriate physician supervision will *reduce* malpractice risks. We believe this for two reasons. First, effective utilization of PAs will allow the physician to concentrate on those medical procedures and judgments that only he can manage. Second, a malpractice suit often results from poor patient rapport rather than negligence per se. When a patient is seen after a considerable wait and then only hurriedly by a harassed physician, the probability of patient dissatisfaction is magnified. Time-motion studies have shown that when a physician's assistant is used waiting periods are reduced, patients receive greater attention from various health professionals, and patient acceptance of the PA has generally been good.[1]

---

1. J. Elliott Dixon, "Ask the Man Who Uses One," in Third Annual Duke Conference on Physician's Assistants, November 12, 1970, available from

An HEW commission on medical malpractice analyzed malpractice in depth. There is increasing interest in making fundamental reforms—e.g., removing the issue from the traditional adversary "fault" framework and using a "no-fault" arbitration approach. The recommendations of the HEW commission have been published.[2]

In summary, we doubt that the use of well-qualified and supervised PAs will increase malpractice risks. We applaud the study of malpractice by the HEW commission, and believe that the utilization of physician's assistants will provide few malpractice issues not already raised by the utilization of nurses and other health professionals. Malpractice questions should not be a deterrent to the development and use of physician's assistants.[3]

CREDENTIALS: ACCREDITATION AND CERTIFICATION

Central to the successful development of the physician's assistant is the need to assure the public of high quality health care. Typically, quality in health education and care is attempted through accreditation, certification, and licensure. Accreditation and certification will be discussed in this section and will be followed by an analysis of alternative licensure schemes.

The National Commission on Accrediting defines accreditation, certification, and licensure as follows: "Accreditation is the process by which an agency or organization evaluates and recognizes a program of study or an institution as meeting certain predetermined qualifications or standards. It shall apply only to institutions and their programs of study or their services."[4] In allied health,

---

the Department of Community Health Services, Duke University, Durham, N.C. pp. 49–62; Eva D. Cohen, *An Evaluation of Policy Related Research on New and Expanded Roles of Health Workers: Executive Summary* (New Haven: Yale University School of Medicine, Office of Regional Activities and Continuing Education, October 1974).

2. U.S. Department of Health, Education and Welfare, *Report of the Secretary's Commission on Medical Malpractice*, pub. no. (OS) 73–88 (Washington, D.C.: U.S. Government Printing Office, 1973).

3. Malpractice insurance is available for the physician's assistant and for the physician who hires him. The Insurance Rating Board has studied the question at the request of the Duke University Physician's Associate Program directors. The board has rendered an official statement that professional liability insurance will be made available to the employing physician at a small additional expense and to the university-trained physician's assistant at a rate of approximately 50 percent of that paid by the employing physician.

4. Study of Accreditation of Selected Health Education Programs, *Commission Report* (Washington, D.C.: National Commission on Accrediting, May 1972).

accreditation usually is undertaken by the AMA in conjunction with the particular occupation's professional association.

Certification is the process by which a nongovernmental agency or association grants recognition to an individual who has met certain predetermined qualifications specified by that agency or association.
Licensure is the process by which an agency of government grants permission to persons meeting predetermined qualifications to engage in a given occupation and/or use a particular title or grants permission to institutions to perform specified functions.[5]

Determining the proper approach to "credentialing" the physician's assistant is difficult because of the widely expressed dissatisfaction with all three of these mechanisms.[6]

The Newman Report

The need for major reform in educational credentialing was urged in a 1971 report on higher education prepared for HEW and funded by the Ford Foundation under the chairmanship of Frank Newman of Stanford University. The report was highly critical of the American "credentials monopoly" and warned:

... when the reliance on education credentials compels individuals to spend tedious hours and years in school against their interest, perpetuates social inequality, gives one group in society unique and arbitrary power over the lives of many, establishes conditions in which people will be dissatisfied and unhappy with their jobs, undermines the educational process, and all this unnecessarily—then the time has come to change these practices. . . . The . . immediate need . . is to break the credentials monopoly by opening up alternative routes to obtaining credentials.[7]

The Newman report also asserted:

In the name of protecting the standards of education, regional and specialized accrediting organizations pressure new institutions to develop faculties, buildings, and educational requirements on the

---

5. Ibid., also Maryland Y. Pennell, John R. Proffitt, and Thomas Hatch, "The Role of Professional Associations in the Regulation of Health Manpower through Accreditation and Certification," *1971 National Health Forum*, pp. 53–78.

6. For example, see David Hapgood, *Diplomaism* (New York: John Brown & Co., 1970); James W. Kuhn, "Would Horatio Alger Need a Degree?," *Saturday Review*, December 19, 1970.

7. Frank Newman, *Report on Higher Education* (to the Secretary of Health, Education and Welfare) (Washington, D.C.: U.S. Government Printing Office, 1971).

pattern of established conventional colleges and universities. More-over, these organizations—dominated by the guilds of each disci-pline—determine the eligibility of these new institutions for public support. We believe that (1) the composition of established accredit-ing organizations should be changed to include representatives of the public interest; and (2) Federal and State governments should reduce their reliance on these established organizations for determining eligibility for Federal support.[8]

The Newman report caused considerable stir in the educational community.

SASHEP

The Study of Accreditation of Selected Health Educa-tional Programs (SASHEP) sponsored by the Council on Medical Education of the AMA, the Association of Schools of Allied Health Professions, and the National Commission on Accrediting began in 1970. Directed by Dr. William K. Selden, the study focused on 15 allied health education programs approved by the AMA as being representative of the gamut of the health professions and services. A series of excellent working papers on various aspects of accreditation have been prepared by the SASHEP staff.[9] The study was completed in 1972, and contained important implications for the accreditation of physician's assistant training programs.

Educational Standards for the PA

The need for standards for the primary care physician's assistant led the AMA's Council on Medical Education Advisory Committee on Education for the Allied Health Professions and Services to form a subcommittee to draft *Essentials of an Approved Educational Program for the Assistant to the Primary Care Physi-cian*. The subcommittee included representatives of the American Academy of Family Physicians (AAFP), American College of Physi-cians (ACP), American Society of Internal Medicine (ASIM), Ameri-can Academy of Pediatrics (AAP), Association of American Medical Colleges (AAMC), and directors of selected PA training programs. A draft of standards for such programs was developed and officially approved by the AAFP, AAP, ACP, ASIM, and the AMA during 1971.[10]

---

8. Ibid., pp. 38, 42.

9. Particularly relevant to this analysis is Karen Grimm, "The Rela-tionship of Accreditation to Voluntary Certification and State Licensure," *SASHEP Staff Working Papers*, vol. 2 (1972).

10. *Essentials of an Approved Educational Program for the Assistant to the Primary Care Physician*, American Medical Association (December 1971) (see pp. 25–33).

Subsequently, a Joint Review Committee for Educational Programs for the Assistant to the Primary Care Physician was organized. Each sponsoring organization has two representatives. The essentials for programs training the assistant to the primary care physician were flexible enough to permit the variety and diversity needed to evaluate the most effective educational approaches and still protect the public from poorly devised and hastily conceived programs. The challenge has been to administer the essentials in a manner which permits flexibility and does not prematurely foreclose fresh and imaginative ideas.

Certification and Proficiency Testing in Allied Health

Amid widespread dissatisfaction with current accreditation and licensure mechanisms, more attention is being placed on development of standards through national certification of health personnel. Central to this effort has been the recognition of the need to develop criteria for proficiency other than the mere completion of an educational program. The Division of Allied Health Manpower of the Bureau of Health Manpower has supported the development of proficiency examinations in physical therapy laboratory technology, radiologic technology, inhalation therapy, and occupational therapy. The number of proficiency tests will undoubtedly increase as more emphasis is placed on satisfactory testing as an alternative to educational credentials.

An HEW *Report on Licensure and Related Health Personnel Credentialing* recommended that the Assistant Secretary for Health and Scientific Affairs explore the feasibility of establishing a national system of certification for those categories of health personnel for which such certification would be appropriate.[11] This recommendation anticipated the creation of an umbrella mechanism at the national (not federal) level for the coordination and direction of certification practices for selected health occupations. The national certification system would establish common policies and practices for certifying agencies; determine the desirability of extending certification to new occupations; carry out studies and make recommendations to improve certifying practices; provide expertise to assist individual agencies in such areas as testing, financing, and logistics; and provide a bridge for coordination with accreditation and licen-

---

11. U.S. Department of Health, Education and Welfare (to the Congress of the United States), *Report on Licensure and Related Health Personnel Credentialing*, HEW pub. no. (ASM) 72–11 (July 28, 1971), p. 73.

sure. HEW has given top priority to studying the feasibility of an umbrella certification system.[12]

National Certification for PAs

In November 1971, the AMA House of Delegates directed its Council on Health Manpower to assume a leadership role in sponsoring a national program for certification of the "Assistant to the Primary Care Physician" who functions as a Type A physician's assistant. National certification was favored to provide geographical mobility for physician's assistants, provide the physician employer with some evidence of competency, and permit greater flexibility than state licensure.

In presenting this proposal to the Federation of State Medical Boards in February 1972, Dr. Malcom C. Todd, chairman of the AMA's Council on Health Manpower, noted that other health occupations such as occupational therapists and medical record librarians certify their own workers at the assistant level. He suggested that physicians exercise the same prerogative with respect to their assistants. Dr. Todd added:

> In the absence of uniform curricula for assistants, the major emphasis of any certification process should be placed on actual job proficiency. If the examination is to be primarily a measure of proficiency, applications should also be accepted from persons who are not graduates of approved programs but who have gained their knowledge and skill through experience and other non-traditional ways. In the past, most written certification examinations have tested book knowledge instead of measuring the proficiency required for the delivery of services and this constitutes a major criticism of professional certification.[13]

Efforts toward national certification moved briskly. In March 1972 the AMA's Council on Health Manpower and the National Board of Medical Examiners began to collaborate on the

---

12. In September 1971, a conference on certification of allied health personnel concluded that an indepth study of certification within the allied health fields was desirable and that the study should be undertaken in cooperation with the allied health professional associations. U.S. Department of Health, Education, and Welfare, *Certification in the Allied Health Professions—Proceedings, Invitational Conference*, publication no. 72–246 (NIH) (Washington, D.C.: U.S. Government Printing Office, 1972). See also Maryland Y. Pennell and David B. Hoover, "Policies for the Development of Credentialing Mechanisms for Health Personnel," *Operation MEDIHC Newsletter* 2, no. 3 (February 1972), published by the National Health Council, New York.

13. Malcolm C. Todd, "Proposed National Certification of Physician's Assistants by Uniform Examinations" (Presented at the Federation of State Medical Boards of the United States, February 4, 1972), p. 8.

development of national certification for physician's assistants. The long-standing experience of the National Board of Medical Examiners in testing made it an ideal organization to undertake the effort.

The important issue of prerequisites to take the national examination was addressed by an advisory committee to the national board. Eligibility for the first national examination given in December 1973 was open to graduates of PA, Medex, and nurse practitioners programs. Eligibility for the 1974 national examination was extended to include health professionals who had functioned in practice as assistants to the primary care physician for at least four years and who met additional criteria.[14]

LICENSURE FOR THE PHYSICIAN'S ASSISTANT?

The physician's assistant has arrived at a time when licensure for all health professions is under heavy attack. Enacted in the early twentieth century to protect the public from quacks and incompetent practitioners, licensure laws now are viewed as unnecessary barriers to educational advance, effective delegation of tasks, and innovation in manpower utilization. Further, they have failed to solve the problems of the incompetent and unethical practitioner.[15]

These conclusions appear in position statements on licensure prepared in 1970 by the American Medical Association and the American Hospital Association and are consistent with the views of most scholars in the field.[16] The *Report on Licensure and Related Health Personnel Credentialing* issued in June 1971 by HEW reached the same conclusion and joined with the previous statements in urging a moratorium on licensure of additional health occupations.[17]

The development of various types of physician's assistants throughout the country has further complicated the issue. Heralded from the inception as a "legally dependent" person who would prac-

---

14. Additional information can be obtained from the National Board of Medical Examiners in Philadelphia.

15. See Edward Forgotson, Charles Bradley, and Martha Ballenger, "Health Services for the Poor—The Manpower Problem: Innovations and the Law," *Wisconsin Law Review* 1970, no. 3 (December 1970):756–89; Arthur Leff, "Medical Devices and Paramedical Personnel: A Preliminary Context for Emerging Problems, *Washington University Law Quarterly* 1967, no. 3 (Summer 1967):332–413.

16. American Medical Association, Council on Health Manpower, *Licensure of Health Occupations* (adopted December 1970); American Hospital Association, Special Committee on Licensure of Health Personnel, *Statement on Licensure of Health Personnel* (approved November 18, 1970).

17. HEW, *Report on Licensure*.

tice only under the "supervision and control" of the physician, the PA has directed attention to the thorny problem of a proper umbrella for the delegation of medical tasks. The National Advisory Commission on Health Manpower concluded in 1967 that, of the many problems presented by the medical licensure laws, the issue of delegation of tasks is the most significant problem requiring resolution.[18] The report noted that such resolution would involve not only the medical profession, but nursing and other allied professions, and would require consideration of the legal regulation and scope of functions of all the occupations which render personal health care.

Nearly everyone opposes licensure of the physician's assistant, but the alternatives to licensure vary. After two years of work, a Duke University task force could not agree on which one of three approaches was superior:

1. to merely codify the authority of the physician to delegate tasks to physician's assistants,
2. to also require prior approval of training programs by a board (such as the state Board of Medical Examiners); or
3. to require submission to the board of a job description of the physician's assistant and the qualifications of the supervising physician.[19]

Some support "institutional" licensure whereby the institution in which the personnel are employed is responsible totally for hiring and firing as well as the quality of care. Professor Nathan Hershey advocates this approach:

> The state hospital licensing agency could establish, with the advice of experts in the health care field, job descriptions for various hospital positions and establish qualifications in terms of education and experience for individuals who would hold these posts. Administrators certainly recognize the fact that although a professional nurse is licensed, her license does not automatically indicate which positions within the hospital she is qualified to fill. Individuals, because of their personal attainment, are selected to fill specific posts. Educational qualifications, based on both formal and in-service programs, along with prior job experience, determine if and how personnel should be employed. One distinct advantage to this

18. *Report of the National Advisory Commission on Health Manpower*, vol. II (Washington, D.C., 1968), p. 332.
19. Martha Ballenger and E. Harvey Estes, *Model Legislation Project for Physician's Assistants* (Durham, N.C.: Duke University, Durham, N.C.: Department of Community Health Sciences, 1969).

scheme is that it would afford the institutional employer wide latitude in utilizing personnel, subject only to the job descriptions. Presumably, it would allow the flexible use of licensed manpower in certain approved jobs.[20]

Others prefer licensure of health teams because of the increasing acceptance of team delivery of patient care. While encouraging a "team" approach, Ruth Roemer notes that the transition from solo practitioners to a system of health care teams is occurring at an uneven rate. She concedes that two systems of regulating health personnel may be needed—one for practitioners to whom patients have direct access and another for practitioners in institutional settings.[21] Subsequently, Ruth Roemer developed 20 different approaches to the licensure question.[22]

THE DELEGATION AMENDMENT—
A FINGER IN THE DIKE

While conceptual approaches are debated, one short run alternative to licensure has received wide acceptance. The AMA, AHA, and HEW all recommend that the states enact amendments to their medical practice acts to codify the right of a physician to delegate tasks to health personnel working under his supervision and control. Although the doctrine of "custom and usage" establishes the authority of physicians to delegate tasks, it does not apply readily to innovations in the utilization of existing health workers or to new types of personnel, such as physician's assistants.[23] At least 37 states have adopted some form of amendment to their medical practice acts.[24]

Most amendments make no attempt to define the tasks or under what situations the tasks may be delegated. Typically, they provide that "any act, task or function" ("services performed" or "services rendered") may be delegated by the physician.[25]

---

20. Nathan Hershey, "An Alternative to Mandatory Licensure of Health Professionals," *Hospital Progress* 50, (March 1969):71–73. For an excellent discussion of institutional licensure see Rick J. Carlson, "Health Manpower Licensing and Emerging Institutional Responsibility for the Quality of Care," *Law & Contemporary Problems* 35, no. 4 (Autumn 1970):849–78.

21. Ruth Roemer, "Licensing and Regulation of Medical and Medical-Related Practitioners in Health Service Teams," *Medical Care* 9, no. 1 (January–February 1971):42–45.

22. Ruth Roemer, "Legal Regulation of Health Manpower in the 1970s: Needs, Objectives, Options, Constraints, and their Trade-Offs," *1971 National Health Forum*.

23. Forgotson, Bradley, and Ballenger, p. 777.

24. See Appendix B. For the AMA recommended language, see p. 113.

25. "Any act, task, or function" (North Carolina); "selected medical tasks" (West Virginia); "services rendered" (Connecticut). The new Washing-

All such delegation amendments require that the acts be performed under the "supervision, control and responsibility" of the licensed physician. The language relating to supervision and control varies in each statute, leaving the legal resolution of this question, should it arise, to the courts on a case by case basis.[26] This is probably wise in light of the small number of physician's assistant graduates to date and the variety of settings in which they practice.

Supervision can take place on at least three levels: (1) over the shoulder, (2) on the premises, and (3) remote with regular monitoring and review. It is quite possible that quality of care with remote supervision can equal care with over the shoulder supervision, if the physician's assistant is well qualified and there is adequate task definition and review. Thus, physician's assistants or nurse practitioners can work at substantial distance from the physician but still be legally "dependent" because their actions are subject to continuous medical review and direction.

Beyond the requirement of supervision and control, several states have followed 1970 California legislation that precludes a person from practicing as a physician's assistant unless he is also a graduate of a program approved by the state board of medical examiners.[27] Prior approval is intended to provide greater uniformity of programs in order to protect the public.

Overregulation—California 1971

Initially, the California statute was heralded as "the nation's most complete and comprehensive 'physician's assistant' law."[28] But proposed rules prepared by the California Board of

---

ton law is unique in defining the physician's assistant as one "who practices medicine to a limited extent," *Washington Acts*, ch. 30 (April 8, 1971). (See pp. 000–000.)

26. The Arkansas statute requires "direct supervision and control," while the Alaska law permits "direct communication, when necessary . . . with the physician . . . either by telephone, or any other immediate method" and requires that "the work of the physician's assistant be regularly reviewed by the physician." The Iowa and New York statutes require physician "supervision and control" but state that this "shall not be construed to necessarily require the personal presence of the supervising physician at the place where services are rendered."

27. *California Business and Professional Code*, Section 2511 (d) (West Supplement, 1971). See also, Appendix B.

28. William J. Curran, "The California 'Physicians' Assistants' Law," *New England Journal of Medicine* 283, no. 23 (December 3, 1970):1274–75. Professor Curran continued: "It goes considerably beyond any other state statute in this new and growing field in providing a firm legal foundation for the development of such programs. It also provides protection to the public by assuring that a responsible state agency is overseeing the program and regulating the entry of qualified, well-trained assistants into practice. . . . On the whole, the Califor-

Medical Examiners on October 25, 1971 were very restrictive and created a considerable controversy. Particularly onerous to many was the requirement that all PA training programs must be two years in length.[29]

Following extensive public hearings, the two year requirement was reduced to "a minimum period of one year . . . spent in residence in full time clinical training with direct patient contact."[30] However, the regulations as finally adopted include a detailed list of tasks that a PA can perform. An approved educational program must include junior college level courses in algebra, sociology, or cultural anthropology and psychology. The regulations provide that the course work of an approved program shall carry academic credit and that, upon completion of the program, the student shall have academic credits equivalent to an associate degree.[31]

Finally, the regulations define supervision as requiring the physician to consult with the PA and the patient before and after the rendering of routine laboratory, screening, and therapeutic procedures.[32] In so doing, the board has sharply limited the effectiveness of the PA in California. The California experience shows the dangers of trying to overregulate a newly emerging health profession at a time when flexibility and innovation are essential.[33]

In other states, such as Washington, prior program approval has proved workable where the state board and medical society appear more flexible and play a significant role in the selection of physician preceptors for the Seattle Medex program. However, no

---

nia law is a basically sound piece of legislation. . . ." But as Professor Curran conceded: "The success of the program in California now depends upon the imagination and good faith of the California Board of Medical Examiners." . . .

29. Mr. Gordon Duffy (chairman of the California State Assembly Health Committee), who introduced the legislation, has been quoted as being very upset with the proposed rules. The board, he said, "apparently did not understand that emphasis should be placed on the requisition of skills not degrees." "Setback for Medex Programs," *Medical World News* 12 (November 19, 1971):83–84.

30. *Regulations of the Physician's Assistant Examining Committee of the Board of Medical Examiners of the State of California*, Chapter 13, Article 15, Section 1379.25 (1971) (see pp. 115–123).

31. Ibid., Section 1379.24. (e).

32. Ibid., Section 1379.22.

33. To assure adequate identification of the PA the California board has proposed the additional regulation: "An assistant . . . shall at all times when rendering medical services wear an identification badge not less than two and one-half inches long on his outer garment which shall in print not less than one-fourth inch in size state the assistant's name and the title 'Assistant to the Primary Care Physician.' A trainee enrolled in an approved education program . . . shall at all times when rendering medical services wear a blue coat. . . ." A specified identification badge is also required for the trainee.

matter how it is administered, prior program approval contains major weaknesses. By requiring practicing physician's assistants to be graduates of approved programs, focus is placed on course content, credits, and degrees. This results in less emphasis on the tasks to be delegated or the situations in which they will be performed. Emphasis is placed on educational inputs rather than practice outputs. Thus, the competence of the PA and the safety of the patient are not necessarily guaranteed.

Prior approval transforms the state board of medical examiners into an accrediting body. Generally, these boards do not accredit medical schools or hospitals and do not have the years of experience in accreditation possessed by the American Medical Association, Association of American Medical Colleges, and the American Hospital Association.

Moreover, an "accrediting" body composed of physicians is less desirable than one with mixed representation from other health fields, hospitals, and the public. State boards of medical examiners naturally tend to be guild-oriented and some have been more inclined to protect the interests of the physician than society. The lack of public representation on health accrediting and licensing bodies has received increasing criticism in recent years, criticism which is consistent with the generally recognized need for a greater consumer voice in the delivery of health care.[34]

Finally, some prior approval statutes, such as California's, apparently require that no reasons be given for program disapproval or revocation. No right of appeal or review is provided. The regulation of an important new health profession must be consistent with the basic principles of due process.[35]

In summary, general delegation statutes are merely an opening-up mechanism to encourage experimentation and innovation. The further development of physician's assistants (particularly their relationship to nurses, physicians, and other health personnel) requires a fundamental reexamination of their scope of practice. Nothing less than a comprehensive reexamination of the "practice of medicine" and the "practice of nursing" is required.

---

34. For example, see William Selden, "Licensing Boards are Archaic," *American Journal of Nursing* 70, no. 1 (January 1970):124–26. For a cogent articulation of additional weaknesses of the prior program approval approach and the advantages of legal flexibility, see Clark C. Havighurst, "Licensure and its Alternatives," The Third Annual Duke Conference on Physician's Assistants, pp. 121–31.

35. See William A. Kaplan, "The Law's View of Professional Power: Courts and the Health Professional Associations," *SASHEP Staff Working Papers*, vol. 2 (1972); William A. Kaplan and J. Philip Hunter, "The Legal Status of the Educational Accrediting Agency: Problems in Judicial Supervision and Governmental Regulation," *Cornell Law Quarterly* 52 (1966):104–31.

DEFINITIONS OF THE PRACTICE
OF MEDICINE AND NURSING

Typically, state medical practice acts provide that no one can "diagnose, operate, treat, or prescribe" unless he is a physician licensed in the state. With two recent exceptions to be discussed,[36] the law has restricted these four words and the practices they represent to the physician. Educators, practitioners, and lawyers, trying to fit dynamic health manpower developments into an archaic legal structure, have been forced to play charades with the law.

The 1955 model Nursing Practice Act prepared by the ANA is an example. After defining the practice of professional nursing,[37] it warns: [this] *shall not be deemed to include acts of diagnosis or prescription of therapeutic or corrective measures"* (emphasis added). Twenty states have enacted nursing practice acts which contain this specific caveat.

One obvious problem with these laws is that "operate, diagnose, treat, and prescribe" are never defined. Although diagnosis has been defined in the literature as "ascertaining a disease or ailment by its symptoms," this simple definition may be difficult to apply in a specific case.[38]

Courts have taken differing views on the meaning of "diagnosis." Some hold that the nurse is properly allowed the responsibility of judging the gravity of symptoms without engaging in

---

36. The Child Health Associate Law enacted in Colorado in 1969 allows the child health associate to "practice pediatrics" and to "prescribe" certain nonnarcotic drugs under very specific restrictions. The new Washington delegation amendment allows a physician's assistant to "practice medicine to a limited extent."

37. The model law defines the "practice of professional nursing" as the "observing, care and counsel of the ill, injured or infirm, or the maintenance of health or prevention of illness of others, or the supervision and teaching of other personnel, or the administration of medications in treatments as prescribed by a licensed physician or licensed dentist; requiring substantial specialized judgment and skill based on knowledge and application of the principles of biological, physical and social science." *Report of the National Advisory Commission on Health Manpower*, vol. II, p. 489.

38. "Consider the nurse in the intensive care unit who is operating [sic] under standing orders. Using this definition, diagnosis would be the selection of one disease from a possibility of diseases suggested by the symptoms. On the other hand, diagnosis would not be a judgment of whether a symptom is present or a judgment of the seriousness of the symptoms. When the nurse judges that the patient exhibits ventricular fibrillation, she is merely observing a symptom not diagnosing the disease suggested. In determining that the patient is suffering a true cardiac arrest, she is exercising judgment as to the seriousness of the symptoms, but she is not ascertaining the nature of the disease." Note, "Acts of Diagnosis by Nurses and the Colorado Professional Nursing Act," *Denver Law Journal* 45 (1968):p. 467. One could reasonably reach the opposite conclusion on these facts.

diagnosis. Others conclude that when a nurse evaluates a symptom and decides that no serious disease is indicated, she is diagnosing. The interpretations of "diagnosis" must be examined in relation to the statutes in which the word appears. Courts may properly attempt a broad definition of "diagnosis" if it appears in a statute which prohibits an unlicensed person from holding himself out as being able to diagnose, treat, operate, or prescribe. On the other hand, public policy has led courts to adopt a more narrow definition of "diagnosis" if acts of judgment are performed by a well-trained nurse.[39]

The uncertainty surrounding diagnosis has been widely recognized in the literature. In their definitive book, *Nursing Practice and the Law*, Lesnik and Anderson attribute this confusion to the fact that "an obligation to observe symptoms and reactions (nursing functions) seems to be intertwined inextricably with diagnosis and the latter generally is acknowledged within the exclusive province of those who practice medicine . . . nevertheless, there is an area with which the nurse is charged, and that area may well be called *nursing diagnosis*" (emphasis added). Lesnik and Anderson note that

> diagnosis involves the utilization of intelligence and interpreting known facts. The decision is the result of the interpretation. Certainly, the utilization of intelligence is an inseparable aspect of the science of diagnosis. Where a decision is made, or should be made, some action must follow. There can be no question that a nurse is required to interpret known facts and make a decision based on them.[40]

In their 1966 article entitled "Clinical Inference in Nursing," Hammond and Kelly concluded that the "inferential or diagnostic task" was central to all nursing practice.[41] They noted that,

---

39. In the landmark California case of *Cooper* v. *National Motor Bearing Company*, 136 Cal. App. 2d 229, 238, 288 P.2d 581, 587 (1955), the court concluded that a nurse, evaluating the seriousness of a symptom, was making an act of diagnosis. The court stated: "A nurse in order to administer first aid properly and effectively must make a sufficient diagnosis to enable her to apply the appropriate remedy. . . . She has been trained, but to a lesser degree than a physician, in the recognition of the symptoms of diseases and injuries. She should be able to diagnose . . . sufficiently to know whether . . . it bears danger signs that should warn her to send the patient to a physician." The court was saying, in essence, that in order to administer *first aid* (generally thought of as *not* the practice of medicine) a nurse was making a diagnosis. That is, a nurse is making a diagnosis when she decides that no serious disease or symptom is indicated and the patient need not see a doctor.

40. Milton J. Lesnik and Bernice E. Anderson, *Nursing Practice and the Law* (Philadelphia: J. B. Lippincott, 1955), p. 265.

41. Hammond, Kelly, Schneider, and Vancini, "Clinical Inference in Nursing," *Nursing Research* 15 (Spring 1966):134–38.

since the time of Florence Nightingale, emphasis has been placed not only on the need to observe but also on how to observe. For years the observational task of the nurse consisted of three activities, namely, observing, recording, and reporting. Hammond and Kelly state:

> more recently the observational function is now conceived to be a process that includes three specific operations: observation—recognition of signs and symptoms presented by the patient; inference- making a judgment about the state of the patient and/or nursing needs of the patient; and decision making—determining the action to be taken that will be of optimal benefit to the patient. Although all three tasks are cognitive functions, the second and third are clearly intellectual in character.[42]

In placing the "inferential or diagnostic task" of the nurse within the boundaries of nursing practice, Hammond and Kelly recognize the need for a distinction "between the functions and responsibilities of the nurse as a diagnostician and the physician as a diagnostician." Their distinction is: "just as the keystone of modern medicine is the identification of disease and its eradication through specifics, the keystone of modern nursing is the determination of a symptom and its alleviation." The need for some distinction is highlighted in the subsequent discussion of the New York Nursing Law[43] and is essential to the development and definition of the role of the physician's assistant.

Graduates of pediatric nurse practitioner programs provide excellent evidence that nurses can assume expanded roles in the area of child health care and can assume many tasks requiring considerable judgment and discretion.[44] These should be recognized as

---

42. A further significant finding in their research is that the inferential decision and action must at times take place in a span of a few minutes or less. The coronary care unit is again an example.

43. See pp. 106–110.

44. In describing his pediatric nurse practitioner program developed at the University of Colorado, Dr. Henry Silver states: "Pediatric Nurse Practitioners are able to give *total care* to more than 75% of all children who come to the field stations, including almost all of the well children (who make up slightly more than one-half of all patients) as well as approximately one-half of the children with illnesses or injuries" (emphasis added). He also notes that nurses "serve in a variety of field stations" and that, in many of these field stations, physicians only visit the station once or twice a week when they see patients with "special problems." He adds: "Nurses always function under the supervision and direction of a physician, even though he may not be physically present at all times." If the Colorado pediatric nurse practitioner is giving "total care" to a group of patients, "diagnosis and treatment" are clearly part of this process. Dr. Silver avoids these words when he states that the nurse will have "taken a complete history, performed a thorough physical examina-

diagnosis and treatment functions. A joint statement of the ANA and the American Academy of Pediatrics, issued in January 1971, dodged the diagnosis question by stating: "The expansion of the nurse's responsibilities should be viewed as increasing the sources from which the nurse gathers data *for making nursing assessments as a basis for diagnosis and action* and thus contribute directly to comprehensive nursing"[45] (emphasis added).

The above discussion about diagnosis could be applied to "operating, treating, and prescribing"—the other traditionally "physician only" functions. Numerous examples of "operating" (starting intravenous fluids or suturing a minor laceration), "treating" (managing common illness), and "prescribing" (completing prescriptions already signed according to standing orders)[46] can be readily found in tasks performed by nurses, and it is clear that physician's assistants will be performing even more of these physicianlike tasks.

In recent years, two state laws (Colorado and Washington) have pierced explicitly the "only-a-physician-can-practice-medicine veil."

Colorado's Child Health Associate Law

The child health associate law enacted in Colorado in 1969 defines a child health associate as "a person who, subject to the limitations provided by this act, *practices pediatrics* as an employee of and under the direction and supervision of a physician whose

---

tion, and make a *tentative assessment and evaluation* with particular emphasis on the differentiation of normal from abnormal findings and a preliminary interpretation of the latter" (emphasis added). Henry Silver, "The Pediatric Nurse Practitioner Program," *Journal of the American Medical Association* 204, no.,4 (April 22, 1968):298–302.

45. "Guidelines on Short-Term Continuing Education Programs for Pediatric Nurse Associates" Joint statement of the American Nurses Association and the American Academy of Pediatrics, January 1971).

46. The use of "standing orders" is another game often played with the law. In effect, standing orders presume to constitute medical direction for the "execution" of medical "decisions" in the physician's absence. Anderson and Lesnik say that "to the extent that orders constitute instructions for cases *already diagnosed*, such orders are valid." However, "a physician may not delegate the authority to diagnose, to treat, or to prescribe. A standing order for treatment of a headache or a cold is illegal since it presupposes a prescription based on diagnosis." Lesnik and Anderson, p. 281. This puts us back on the semantic merry-go-round. The standing orders mechanism should be valuable in setting the appropriate limits of a PAs function. Standing orders can be readily amended by the physician as needed. The HEW definition of a physician's assistant states: "He may, on the basis of standing orders, treat a defined range of medical conditions and may provide emergency care in keeping with his training and as permitted by his supervising physician. Although effective supervision is required, it need not in all cases be face-to-face" (see p. 22).

practice to a substantial extent is in pediatrics" (emphasis added). However, the act limits the child health associate "to practice only in the professional office of the employing physician and only during the time when the employing physician . . . is directly and personally available." The law sets another important precedent by explicitly permitting the child health associate to "prescribe drugs, except narcotic drugs," which have been approved by an Advisory Committee.[47]

Although the child health associate law has been severely criticized because of the strict requirement of personal presence, supervision, and control, it does specifically allow the practice of a segment of medicine by this new professional and the prescribing of drugs.[48]

Washington's Physician's Assistant Law

In 1971, the state of Washington enacted a statute that permits a "physician's assistant to *practice medicine* to a limited extent under the supervision and control of a physician" (emphasis added). The statute also provides that supervision and control "shall not be construed to necessarily require the personal presence of the supervising physician at the place where services are rendered."

The primary restriction is the requirement that the PA be a graduate of a program approved by the state board of medical examiners "who shall adopt rules and regulations governing the extent to which physician's assistants may practice medicine. . . ." The thorny problem of defining appropriate limits to the scope of practice of the physician's assistant is placed with the state board of medical examiners. The board reviews the competence of the individual physician, as well as the competence and job description of the physician's assistant. The Washington law is an important advance

---

47. The law further states that "a child health associate shall not perform any operative or any cutting procedure or engage in the treatment of fractures . . . " (see pp. 125–132).

48. Professor William Curran has called the Colorado law "an excellent model of what should *not* be done with any licensed group of professionals" and concludes that "the Colorado legislature, the board of medical examiners and the organized medical groups seem to have enacted a high price for granting licensure to this new group of health professionals." William J. Curran, "New Paramedical Personnel—To License or Not to License," *New England Journal of Medicine* 282, no. 19 (May 7, 1970):1085–86. In contrast, Dr. Henry Silver believes that the law "is a progressive, pioneering and innovative legislative act that should serve as a guide in regulating the practice of other categories of new allied health professionals." Henry K. Silver, "New Allied Health Professionals: Implications of the Colorado Child Health Associate Law," *New England Journal of Medicine* 284, no. 6 (February 11, 1971):304–07.

because it explicitly recognizes that much of what a physician's assistant does is the practice of medicine.

These legal developments may help to whittle away the clichés that have confused scope of practice issues. The September 27, 1971 issue of *JAMA* contained an unsigned editorial on physician's assistants which cautioned: "State laws provide that only a licensed physician may engage in the practice of medicine and that it is illegal for a physician to delegate the practice of medicine to a person who is not a licensed physician." The article continued: "On the other hand, it is entirely legal for a physician to use a technician as his 'hands' in work which does not involve a delegation of 'medical discretion.'"[49]

Such statements are incorrect and out of date in light of recent legal developments and the recognition that the practice of medicine increasingly overlaps other professions.[50] In a 1970 report entitled "Medicine and Nursing Care in the 1970s—A Position Statement," the AMA Committee on Nursing concluded that: "as there is marked overlap in the technical areas common to medical and nursing practice, the same act may be clearly the practice of medicine when performed by a physician and the practice of nursing when performed by a nurse."[51] This description begs the basic need to:

1. recognize certain diagnosing, treating, operating, and prescribing functions by physician's assistants and nurses; and
2. properly delineate the difference between the tasks that can be performed by physician's assistants and nurses from those which should be reserved for the physician.[52]

49. Editorial, "The Medical Manpower Shortage," *Journal of the American Medical Association* 217, no. 13 (September 27, 1971):1857–59.

50. The 1970 AMA report on licensure was surprisingly candid when, in urging states to enact general delegation amendments, it said: "Such an amendment would codify the physician's right to delegate, as well as the *delagatee's right to participate in the practice of medicine*" (emphasis added). *Licensure of Health Occupations*, p. 6 (see p. 113).

An example of the misunderstanding of delegation appears in the August 1971, issue of *Connecticut Medicine*. The Connecticut State Medical Society opposed the AMA-suggested amendment concluding: "In effect, the bill authorizes physician's assistants to practice medicine without a license, provided that they practice under the supervision of a physician. This will establish a most dangerous precedent, and is not at all equivalent to authorizing Doctors of Medicine to utilize the services of qualified assistants in carrying on and expanding the scope of their medical practices." "Forewarned is Forearmed: Governor Signs Physician's Assistant Bill," *Connecticut Medicine* 35, no. 2 (August 1971): 78–80.

51. American Medical Association, Committee on Nursing, "Medicine and Nursing in the 1970's—A Position Statement," *Journal of the American Medical Association* 213, no. 11 (September 14, 1970):1881–83.

52. A report of the HEW secretary's Committee to Study Extended Roles for Nurses examines the increasing scope of nursing in three areas: primary

INDEPENDENCE, DEPENDENCE, AND EXPANDING ROLES

The dependence-independence issue permeates all discussion of the PA's scope of practice. By assuming a legally dependent position, physician's assistants are able to assume far more responsibility than if they attempt to work independently. Some implications of this concept have been discussed previously[53] (see pp. 14–15).

As the above analysis reveals, the delegation amendments enacted in 1971 do not contain detailed guidelines on this issue, but foster dependence through flexible supervision and control provisions. Under these laws, the physician's assistants are authorized to make independent judgments as they "render service," in some instances, geographically removed from the physician.

However, Oregon has taken a restrictive legislative approach. Its law provides: "A physician's assistant *shall not exercise independent judgment* in determining and prescribing treatment except in life-threatening emergencies"[54] (emphasis added). If this provision is followed literally, it is difficult to imagine a broadly trained "Type A" physician's assistant finding employment in Oregon.

Another aspect of dependence is the method of charging patients for services performed by the physician's assistant. Only two

---

care, acute care, and long term care. The report outlines functions in each area for which nurses are: solely responsible; share responsibility with the physician; and could be prepared to assume further responsibility. It recognizes the need for legal change, but provides no solutions and merely states that: "In this period of rapid transition, the identical procedure performed on a patient may be the practice of medicine when carried out by a physician or the practice of professional nursing when carried out by a nurse." Although the report is a good doctor-nurse model of overlapping functions, it does not address the roles of other allied health workers or physician's assistants. HEW, Secretary's Committee Report, *Extending the Scope of Nursing Practice*, pub. no. 0–720–301 (Washington, D.C.: U.S. Government Printing Office, 1972); reprinted in *Nursing Outlook* 20, no. 1 (January 1972):46–52.

53. Lesnik and Anderson aptly state: "One of the great difficulties inherent in analytical evaluation of nursing functions has been the reluctance of some professionals to ascribe to professional nursing any authority for the independent performance of any act. Historically, the primary function of nursing was assistance, but the process of gradual assumption by professional nurses of many other functions was inevitable. Without doubt, part of nursing involves the application and the execution of legal standing medical orders and these functions are dependent ones, since performance is contingent upon direction or supervision. But it is widely recognized that this is not the whole of nursing practice." Indeed, they assert that "the overwhelming number of functions and the majority of areas of control involve obligations of performance independent of medical orders." Lesnik and Anderson, p. 261.

54. 1971 Oregon Acts, Chapter 649, Section 3 (3) (enacted June 30, 1971).

state laws contain provisions dealing explicitly with compensation. The Wisconsin statute provides that "a physician's assistant may not be self-employed" and the Illinois law states that "physician's assistants may not bill patients or in any way charge for services but shall work under the direction of the physician. . . ."[55]

In contrast to the PA's legally dependent and flexible status, organized nursing has struggled to define its own independent function. In some cases, this has operated to the detriment of expanding the nurse's role. The striving for an "independent" function and the quest for an enlarged role which includes many medical acts (of diagnosis and treatment) will be regarded by many as mutually exclusive. Certainly, the public is more willing to accept the performance of medical tasks by PAs and nurses if they are assured of adequate physician supervision, control, and responsibility.[56] Unless the scope of practice is precisely defined, role enlargement and independence may work at cross purposes, as the following New York case vividly shows.

A CASE STUDY OF CONFLICT—
NEW YORK 1971

Independence Defeated

The complex problems of scope of practice, independence-dependence, and supervision and control were raised during the controversy over proposed Senate Bill 1918 which was designed to change the New York State Nursing Practice Act.[57] In lieu of the old definition, the New York State Nurses Association proposed:

> The practice of the profession of nursing as a registered professional nurse is defined as *diagnosing and treating human responses* to actual or potential health problems through such services as case finding, health teaching, health counseling, and provision of care supportive to or restorative of life and well being and *executing medical regimens prescribed* by a licensed or otherwise legally authorized physician or dentist. (Emphasis added.)

---

55. Wisconsin Assembly Bill (April 15, 1971), p. 707; Illinois House Bill (January 26, 1971), p. 203.

56. Dr. Eugene Stead of Duke University has said succinctly: "The physician's assistant can have independence at a low level of performance, or he can accept dependence and achieve a high level of performance." Eugene A. Stead, "Dependence vs. Independence and its Relationship to the Professional Physician's Assistant," Third Annual Duke Conference on Physician's Assistants, p. 101.

57. New York State Senate Bill 1918 (1971).

The official bulletin of the New York State Nurses Association stated in February 1971: "The intent of the bill is to clearly delineate the elements of the nursing process and to specify the independence of the *nursing* function."[58] The bulletin said that the old Nursing Practice Act is both obsolete and circular in nature and fails to recognize the nurses' role in the increasingly significant area of health maintenance and teaching. The bulletin continued:

> The change proposed would in no way infringe upon the inter-dependent and collaborative relationship between the physician and the nurse, but, would simply specify the nurses' authority to diagnose *nursing* needs and administer to those needs through such services as case finding, health teaching, health counseling, and provision of supportive and restorative nursing services or, in other words, to *practice nursing.*
>
> Inclusion within the law of the diagnostic function would authorize the nurse practitioner to make nursing diagnoses not medical diagnoses. Whereas the diagnosing function as an intellectual process is central to the practice of any number of professionals, including medicine and nursing, the *focus* of this function varies among these professions. For example, the focus in medicine is the nature and degree of pathology or deviation from normalcy; within nursing the focus is the *individual's response* to an actual or potential health problem and the nursing needs arising from such responses.[59]

Unfortunately, the law contained no definitions of diagnosis and treatment and thus did not make these distinctions.

Having convinced the legislators that their intent was to define their own role and not usurp the practice of the physician, the law was passed by both houses. However, Governor Rockefeller vetoed it in July 1971. In his memorandum explaining the veto, the governor acknowledged that it was time to modernize the Nursing Practice Act as it was no longer consistent with modern health practice. But in his view the new definition "failed to maintain a responsible distinction between the professions of medicine and nursing commensurate with the respective training and experience of both professions."[60]

The veto, which was strongly supported by the New York

---

58. New York State Nurses Association Legislative Bulletin, no. 4 (February 16, 1971), p. 1.
59. The nursing bulletin expressed criticism of organized medicine asserting: "Medicine views the nurse as a *physician's* assistant; nursing views the nurse as the *patient's* assistant."
60. Governor Nelson Rockefeller, memorandum filed with Senate Bill 1918 (July 7, 1971).

State Medical Society, stated: "The definition of the practice of nursing contained in the above legislation does not accurately reflect the legitimate nursing function. Indeed, the definition is subject to an interpretation *which would result in nurses being authorized as a practical matter to practice medicine*"[61] (emphasis added). Thus, with the utterance of that tired cliché, the bill was defeated.

The response of the New York State Nurses Association was swift and emotional. The association stated,

> Echoing the myopic positions of the Medical Society of the State of New York and the Hospital Association of New York State, the Governor's statement reflects a total lack of understanding of the essential nature of nursing practice and the legitimate role of the nursing profession. Nursing is viewed *not* as a distinct area of professional practice, but simply as a component of the practice of medicine. This view, obviously, gives rise to the demand that the definition of nursing reflect the nursing practitioners' *dependence* on the physician. NYSNA's proposed definition in no way met this demand. On the contrary, for the first time in the history of licensure for nursing, it clearly stated the independence of the nursing function. It was this factor and *this* factor *alone*, which elicited the Medical Society's opposition.

The nurses association bulletin continued: "Throughout the legislative session the Medical Society advised NYSNA that it would accept NYSNA's proposed definition *providing* that the phrase 'under the supervision of the physician' were added. *Because of our belief that nursing is an independent and distinct profession, such a compromise was totally unacceptable*"[62] (emphasis added).

Dependence Approved

Paralleling these developments, the New York legislature passed and the governor signed a law to authorize the practice of "physician's associates" and "specialist's assistants."[63] In discussing

---

61. Ibid.
62. Letter from Veronica M. Driscoll, Executive Director of the NYSNA, to all NYSNA members and groups concerned with NYSNA's proposed definition of nursing, July 8, 1971.
63. The law provides that the physician's associate must be a graduate of a program approved by the board of medical examiners and "may perform medical services but only under the supervision of a physician and only when such acts and duties as are assigned to him are within the scope of practice of such supervising physician." The specialist's assistant "may perform medical services, but only when under the supervision of a physician and only when such acts and duties as are assigned to him are related to the designated medical specialty for which he is registered and are within the scope of practice of a supervising physician." New York Public Health Law, Section 6532 (enacted in Senate Bill 5703, July 6, 1971).

relationships between the "physician's associate" and other health professions, the governor stated:

obviously if a physician's associate or a specialist's assistant were precluded from doing anything which nurses or other health professionals are authorized to do, there would be little else left for them. While physician's associates and specialist's assistants are not intended to in any way replace existing health professions, they necessarily will perform many of the same duties. I am sure that the Health Department can clarify any confusion which might exist by appropriate administrative regulation.[64]

The complex issue of overlapping areas of practice has thus been turned over to the state health department for resolution through regulation. To this, the New York State Nurses Association responded: "The Health Department's support of a system of institutional licensure is well known—it is clear that the first step towards such a system has been taken by the State of New York. Prospects for improved health care appear grim indeed."[65] The letter of July 13th from the president of the New York State Nurses Association, Evelyn M. Peck, to Governor Rockefeller, displays the bitterness felt by organized nursing toward the governor and organized medicine in the state of New York (see pp. 54–55).

NEW YORK REVISITED—1972

Undaunted by the 1971 defeat, the New York State Nurses Association reintroduced Senate Bill 8274 in 1972. The bill redefined nursing as in 1971, but contained several important additions. It was passed by both houses and was signed into law by Governor Rockefeller on March 15, 1972. The enactment of the law received raves from the NYSNA. A news release quotes Evelyn M. Peck, president of the NYSNA:

Enactment of this definition is a landmark achievement; nursing's unique and historic function has finally been acknowledged and legitimized. The bill which has been acclaimed by nursing organizations throughout the country, will undoubtedly serve as a national model for nursing licensure laws. Its enactment comes at a crucial point . . . the public has demanded reorganization of the health care delivery system and the nursing profession has demonstrated its willingness and ability to respond to that mandate.

---

64. Governor Nelson Rockefeller, memorandum filed with Senate Bill 7075 (July 6, 1971).
65. Letter from Veronica M. Driscoll, p. 1.

Hildegard Peplau, president of the ANA, added: "In signing into law the New York State Nurses Practice Act of 1972, Governor Rockefeller has promoted 'a giant step' in the improvement of health care." Miss Peplau noted that

> nurses have said, for a long time that nursing is different from and complementary to medicine. The Nurse Practice Act gives impetus to the developing partnership in health care of physicians and nurses. The American Nurses Association commends the nurses of New York State for bringing about this historic turning point in the advancement of nursing and health care. Nurses of the other 49 states appreciate their efforts, I'm sure, in this important accomplishment.

Two significant additions to the 1971 bill apparently made the 1972 version acceptable to organized medicine and to the governor of New York. First, the 1972 bill defines "diagnosing," "treating," and "human responses."[66] These definitions try to make it clear that the "nursing diagnosing" referred to in bill 8274 is distinct from "medical diagnosing." Second, the bill provides that "a nursing regimen shall be consistent with and shall not vary any existing medical regimen." Also "nothing in this article shall be construed to confer the authority to practice medicine or dentistry." This language, coupled with the statement in bill 8274 that the practice of nursing shall include executing medical regimens prescribed by a licensed physician, insure the continued dependence of the nurse on the physician when performing medical tasks. Organized medicine and the governor were thereby able to endorse the bill.

CARRYING OUT THE ORDER—
A PAPER TIGER?

Eleanor C. Lambertsen, dean of the Cornell–New York Hospital School of Nursing, focused attention on this issue when she noted that: "Today's nurse does recognize that comparable technologies or

---

66. The bill provides: (1) " 'Diagnosing' in the context of nursing practice means that identification of and discrimination between physical and psychosocial signs and symptoms essential to effective execution and management of the nursing regimen. Such diagnostic privilege is distinct from a medical diagnosis. (2) " 'Treating' means selection and performance of those therapeutic measures essential to the effective execution and management of the nursing regimen, and execution of any prescribed medical regimen. (3) " 'Human responses' means those signs, symptoms and processes which denote the individual's interaction with an actual or potential health problem." New York State Senate Bill 8274 (1972). (See pp. 133–135).

therapeutics may be performed by the nurse as well as the physician's assistant. *Not who does what, but who prescribes and who delegates to whom are at issue*"[67] (emphasis added).

An official position paper entitled "The New York State Nurses Association's Statement on the Physician's Associate and Specialist's Assistant," adopted by the NYSNA Board of Directors on January 31, 1972, focused on the orders issue. The position paper states:

> The physician's associate or specialist's assistant is not a substitute for the physician. The association recognizes the right of the medical profession to determine those medical acts which may be safely delegated to physician's assistants. Similarly, as an independent profession, nursing reserves the right to determine from whom it shall accept delegation. Hence, nursing practitioners shall continue to execute those medical regimens prescribed only by a licensed or otherwise legally authorized physician or dentist. In view of the original intent of the physician's assistant role, i.e., to increase the availability of medical services to the public, the association questions the rationale for consideration of assigning the assistant to write medical orders. It would appear that such utilization unnecessarily limits the assistant's involvement in direct services to patients. However, if the medical profession deems it appropriate to assign to the physician's assistant the task of writing medical orders, then the association believes it appropriate for the physician's assistant to also carry out those orders.

In institutional or group practice settings, it is apparent that orders delegated by a physician (standing orders or otherwise) will be carried out by both physician's assistants and nurses. Suppose that a physician, when making patient rounds and accompanied by his physician's assistant, prescribes the patient's medical regimen for the day. The PA returns later in the day and finds a change in the condition of the patient. He describes his findings to his physician by telephone and receives in turn orders to modify the treatment regimen. The orders are written into the chart to be countersigned at a later time by the physician. The PA will certainly carry out many orders himself, but some of the physician's orders may have to be carried out by the nurse.

We believe that this sequence is likely to be repeated often in hospital practice. Nursing should be legitimately concerned about the source of all orders and the impact of carrying them out. Such is

---

67. Eleanor C. Lambertsen, "Nursing: Not quite M.D., More Than P.A.," *Hospitals, JAHA* 45, no. 23 (December 1, 1971), p. 76.

the basis of safe nursing care. On the other hand, it would be unfortunate indeed if nursing (as expressed in the NYSNA statement, for example) were to be so concerned as to refuse to carry out a physician's orders when written by a PA.

Summing Up

At a time when the entire licensure scheme for regulating health personnel is under widespread attack as being archaic, inefficient, and destructive of change, a variety of delegation amendments to state medical practice acts have been enacted as a direct result of the physician's assistant movement. By being willing to remain legally dependent, accept delegation from physicians, and work under the supervision and control of the physician, physician's assistants are now able to function under broad and flexible legal umbrellas that allow them to perform to their capacity.

Despite the flexibility of the delegation amendments and the rapidity with which they have been adopted, they represent merely a short term solution to the scope of practice problem. Some of the delegation amendments are poorly drawn and contain unnecessary and restrictive requirements of prior program approval by boards of medical examiners that are not equipped to discharge these functions. More fundamentally, they do not come to grips with the underlying need to reexamine the definitions of scope of practice of medicine, nursing, and related health professions. Certainly the physician's assistant, the nurse, and other health professionals are performing tasks that come under the traditional medical rubric of diagnose, operate, treat, and prescribe. We need new definitions that will recognize these decisionmaking judgments and yet delineate clearly those tasks that can only be performed by a physician and should not be delegated. These definitions should be consistent with national efforts to develop certification of proficiency for various types of physician's assistants and nurse practitioners.

Conclusions and Recommendations
for Licensure of Health Occupations*

As noted previously, limitations, and shortcomings in present credentialing mechanisms for health professions and occupations are generally acknowledged. Some of these shortcomings appear to be susceptible immediately to correction while others may be only partially alleviated on a short term basis through modifications in present credentialing systems.

To effect such immediate, short term alleviations, the Council on Health Manpower and the board *recommend:*

(a) That state legislatures be urged to amend state medical practice acts to remove any barriers to increased delegation of tasks to allied health personnel by physicians.

Such an amendment might be phrased as follows: "Nothing in this article shall be so construed as to prohibit service rendered by a physician's trained assistant, a registered nurse, or a licensed practical nurse if such service is rendered under the supervision, control, and responsibility of a licensed physician."

The majority of existing state medical practice acts do not define the practice of medicine in terms of specific functions. However, the amendment of medical practice acts as suggested above would codify the physician's recognized right to delegate patient care functions to competent personnel consistent with the patient's welfare, as well as the delegatee's right to participate in the practice of medicine, and might serve to reassure and encourage physicians to innovate in the use of manpower.

---

*Taken from "Licensure of Health Occupations," prepared by the AMA Council on Health Manpower. Adopted by the AMA House of Delegates, December 1970.

California Board of Medical Examiners Regulations on the Physician's Assistant*

CHAPTER 13

Article 15—Physician's Assistants

Section 1379. *Physician's Assistants Defined.* For purposes of this article, physician's assistants within the meaning of article 18, chapter 5 of the Business and Professions Code are divided into two classifications as follows:

(1) Assistant to the primary care physician; and
(2) Assistant to the specialist physician.

Section 1379.1. *Approval of Educational Programs; Applications.* Educational programs for instruction of an assistant to the primary care physician and assistant to the specialist physician must be approved by the board and shall submit applications for approval on forms provided by said board.

Section 1379.20 *Definition of Assistant to the Primary Care Physician.* For purposes of this article, an assistant to the primary care physician means a person who is a graduate of an approved program of instruction in primary health care, who has passed a certification examination administered by the board, and is approved by the board to perform direct patient care services under the supervision of a primary care physician or physicians approved by the board to supervise such an assistant.

Section 1379.21. *Definition of Primary Care Physician.* For purposes of this article, a primary care physician is a physician,

---

*Prepared by the Physician's Assistant Examining Committee of the California Board of Medical Examiners, December 1971.

approved by the board to supervise a particular assistant to the primary care physician, who evaluates his patients' total health care needs and who accepts initial and continuing responsibility therefore.

Section 1379.22. *Definition of Supervision.* Supervision of an assistant to the primary care physician within the meaning of this article refers to the responsibility of the primary care physician to review findings of the history and physical examination permitted by section 1379.23 (a) and all follow-up physical examinations with said assistant together with the patient at the time of completion of such history and physical examination or follow-up examination and to consult with said assistant and patient before and after the rendering of routine laboratory and screening techniques and therapeutic procedures as described in section 1379.23 (b) (c) and (e), excepting where the rendering of routine laboratory and screening techniques are part of the history and physical examination or follow-up examination performed. The foregoing requirement of the primary care physician to review findings of the history and physical examinations and consultation before the rendering of routine laboratory and screening techniques and therapeutic procedures, shall not apply when the assistant to the primary care physician is attending a patient in a life-threatening emergency pending the arrival of the primary care physician, nor is the presence of the primary care physician necessary when said assistant attends the chronically ill patient at home in the nursing home or extended care facility for the sole purpose of collection of data for the information and consideration of the approved supervising physician.

Section 1379.23. *Tasks Performable by an Assistant to the Primary Care Physician.* An assistant to the primary care physician should be able to perform, under the responsibility and supervision of the primary care physician, selected diagnostic and therapeutic tasks in each of the five major clinical disciplines (medicine, surgery, pediatrics, psychiatry, and obstetrics).

Specifically and by way of limitation, an assistant to the primary care physician should be able to:

(a) Take a complete, detailed and accurate history; perform a complete physical examination, when appropriate, excluding pelvic and endoscopic examination; and record and present pertinent data in a manner meaningful to the primary care physician.

(b) Perform and/or assist in the performance of the following routine laboratory and screening techniques:

   1. The drawing of venous blood and the routine examination of the blood.
   2. Catheterization and the routine urinalysis.

3. Nasogastric intubation and gastric lavage.
4. The collection of and the examination of the stool.
5. The taking of cultures.
6. The performance and reading of skin tests.
7. The performance of pulmonary function tests excluding endoscopic procedures.
8. The performance of tonometry.
9. The performance of audiometry.
10. The taking of EKG tracings.

(c) Perform the following routine therapeutic procedures:
1. Injections.
2. Immunizations.
3. Debridement, suture, and care of superficial wounds.
4. Debridement of minor superficial burns.
5. Removal of foreign bodies from the skin.
6. Removal of sutures.
7. Removal of impacted cerumen.
8. Subcutaneous local anesthesia, excluding any nerve blocks.
9. Anterior nasal packing for epistaxis.
10. Strapping, casting, and splinting of sprains.
11. Removal of cast.
12. Application of traction.
13. Application of physical therapy modalities.
14. Incision and drainage of superficial skin infections.

(d) Recognize and evaluate situations which call for immediate attention of the primary care physician and institute, when necessary, treatment procedures essential for the life of the patient.

(e) Instruct and counsel patients regarding matters pertaining to their physical and mental health, such as diets, social habits, family planning, normal growth and development, aging, and understanding of and long term management of their disease.

(f) Assist the primary care physician in the hospital setting by arranging hospital admissions under the immediate direction of said physician; by accompanying the primary care physician in his rounds and recording physician's patient progress notes; by accurately and appropriately transcribing and/or executing specific orders at the direction of the primary care physician; by compiling and recording detailed narrative case summaries; by completing forms pertinent to the patient's medical record.

(g) Assist the primary care physician in the office in the ordering of drugs and supplies, in the keeping of records, and in the upkeep of equipment.

(h)   Assist the primary care physician in providing services to patients requiring continuing care (home, nursing home, extended care facilities, etc.) including the review of treatment and therapy plans.

(i)   Facilitate the primary care physician's referral of patients to the appropriate health facilities, agencies and resources of the community.

An assistant to the primary care physician should have an understanding of the socioeconomics of medicine, of the roles of various health personnel, and of the ethics and laws under which medicine is practiced and governed.

In addition to the tasks performable listed herein as assistant to the primary care physician may be permitted to perform under supervision of the primary care physician such other tasks except those expressly excluded herein in which adequate training and proficiency can be demonstrated in a manner satisfactory to the board.

Section 1379.24. *General Requirements of an Educational Program for an Assistant to the Primary Care Physician.* An educational program for instruction of an assistant to the primary care physician shall meet the following general requirements, as well as specific curriculum requirements set forth herein, for approval:

(a)   The program shall establish the need for a theoretical and clinical training program graduating an assistant to the primary care physician complementary to the effective delivery of medical services in primary health care.

(b)   Candidates for admission shall have successfully completed an approved high school course of study or have passed a standard equivalency test.
Prior clinical experience in direct patient contact is recommended for each candidate.

(c)   The educational program shall be established in educational institutions approved by the board which meet the standards of the Western Association of Schools and Colleges, or any accrediting agency recognized by the National Commission on Accrediting, and which are affiliated with board-approved clinical facilities associated with a medical school approved by the board.

(d)   The educational program shall develop an evaluation mechanism satisfactory to the board to determine the effectiveness of its theoretical and clinical program compatible with statewide standards, the results of which must be made available to the board annually.

(e)   Course work shall carry academic credit. Upon successful completion of the educational program, the student shall have academic credits for the courses taken of at least the equivalent of the associate of arts or science degree.

(f)   The educational program shall establish equivalency and proficiency testing and other mechanisms whereby full academic credit is given for past education and experience in the courses of the curriculum required in section 1379.25 herein.

(g)   The director of the clinical educational program must be a physician licensed to practice in the state of California who holds a faculty appointment at the educational institution.

(h)   Instructors in the theoretical program and clinical training program shall be competent in their respective fields of instruction and clinical training and be properly qualified.

(i)   The educational program shall establish a definitive candidate selection procedure satisfactory to the board.

(j)   The number of students enrolled in the theoretical program should not exceed the number that can be clinically supervised and trained.

(k)   The educational program shall establish resources for continued operation of the training program through regular budgets, gifts, or endowments.

(l)   The educational program shall require a three month preceptorship for each student in the outpatient practice of a primary care physician as the final part of the educational program.

(m)   The educational program shall establish a continuing clinical educational program for assistants to the primary care physician.

(n)   An educational program approved by the board as meeting the general educational requirements above and specific curriculum requirements established in this article for educational programs for an assistant to the primary care physician shall notify the board whenever a change occurs in the directorship of the educational program or when major modifications in the curriculum are anticipated.

(o)   Failure of an educational program to continue compliance with the foregoing general requirements and the specific curriculum requirements of section 1379.25 herein subsequent to approval by the board may result in the board withdrawing said approval.

Section 1379.25. *Curriculum Requirements of an Educational Program for an Assistant to the Primary Care Physician.* The curriculum of an educational program for instruction of an assistant to the primary care physician shall include adequate theoretical instruction in the following:

Basic Educational Core
Physics (to the extent necessary to the practice of medicine)
Chemistry (to the extent necessary to the practice of medicine)

Basic Health Science Core

Mathematics including algebra
English
Anatomy and physiology
Microbiology
Sociology or cultural anthropology
Psychology
(All at the junior college level or its equivalent)

The curriculum of an educational program shall also include adequate theoretical and clinical instruction which must include direct patient contact where appropriate, in the following:

Clinical Science Core

Community health and preventive medicine
Mental health
History taking and physical diagnosis
Management of common diseases (acute, chronic, and emergent) including first aid
Concepts in medicine and surgery, such as:
  growth and development
  nutrition
  aging
  infection and asepsis
  allergy and sensitivity
  tissue healing and repair
  oncology
Common laboratory and screening techniques
Common medical and surgical procedures
Therapeutics, including pharmacology
Medical terminology

Medical ethics and law
Medical socioeconomics
Counseling techniques and interpersonal dynamics

Pursuant to the provisions of section 1379.24(f) herein, the foregoing curriculum can be challenged for full academic credit through equivalency and proficiency testing and other mechanisms, except that no student shall be graduated unless a minimum period of one year is spent in residence in full time clinical training with direct patient contact.

1379.40. *Definition of Assistant to the Specialist Physician.* An assistant to the specialist physician means a person who is a graduate of an approved program for instruction in a recognized clinical specialty who has passed a certification examination administered by the board and is approved by the board to perform direct patient care services in said specialty under the supervision of a physician or physicians approved by the board to supervise such assistant.

1379.41. *General Requirements of an Educational Program as an Assistant to the Specialist Physician.* An educational program for instruction as an assistant to the specialist physician in any recognized clinical specialty shall meet the following general requirements, as well as specific curriculum requirements for the particular specialty more specifically set forth herein, for approval:

(a) The program shall establish that its theoretical and clinical training program produces an assistant to the specialist physician necessary to the effective delivery of medical services within that specialty.

(b) Candidates for admission shall have successfully completed an approved high school course of study or have passed a standard equivalency test. Prior clinical experience in direct patient contact is recommended for each candidate.

(c) The educational program shall be established in educational institutions approved by the board which meet the standards of the Western Association of Schools and Colleges or any accrediting agency recognized by the National Commission on Accrediting and which are affiliated with board approved clinical facilities associated with a medical school approved by the board.

(d) The educational program shall develop an evaluation mechanism satisfactory to the board to determine the effectiveness of its theoretical and clinical program compatible with statewide standards, the results of which must be made available to the board annually.

(e) Course work shall carry academic credit. Upon successful completion of the theoretical and clinical program the student shall receive an associate of arts or science degree.

(f) The educational program shall establish equivalency and proficiency testing and other mechanisms whereby full academic credit is given for past education and experience in the courses of the curriculum required for the particular specialty, more specifically set forth herein.

(g) The director of the educational program must be a licensed physician who is certified as or eligible to be a member of the American board for the particular specialty and who holds a faculty appointment at the educational institution.

(h) Instructors in the theoretical program and clinical training program shall be competent in their respective fields of instruction and clinical training and be properly qualified.

(i) The educational program shall establish a definitive candidate selection procedure satisfactory to the board.

(j) The number of students enrolled in the theoretical program should not exceed the number that can be clinically supervised and trained.

(k) The educational program shall establish resources for continued operation of the training program through regular budgets, gifts or endowments.

(l) The educational program shall have an elective period, preferably near the end of the program, to permit the student to gain knowledge of subjects which pertain to the clinical specialty and the student's particular intended employment thereof.

(m) The educational program shall establish a continuing clinical educational program for health care associates in the particular specialty.

(n) An educational program approved by the board as meeting the general requirements above and specific curriculum requirements established in this article for the particular curriculum specialty shall notify the board whenever a change occurs in the directorship of the educational program or when major modifications in the curriculum are anticipated.

(o) Failure of an educational program to continue compliance with the foregoing general requirements and the specific curriculum requirements for the particular specialty set forth herein subsequent to approval by the board may result in the board withdrawing said approval.

Section 1379.60. *Curriculum Requirements of an Educational Program for Assistant to the Orthopaedic Physician.* An approved educational program for instruction of an assistant to the orthopaedic physician must extend over a period of two academic years and the total number of hours of all courses shall consist of a minimum of 62 semester units. The curriculum shall provide for adequate instruction in the general education requirements for an associate of arts or science degree in the following:

Health Careers

Human anatomy and physiology
Advanced safety service
Introductory microbiology
Psychology
Sociology
Orientation to patient care and staff relationships

Orthopaedic Assisting

Patient service and emergency room technique
Orientation to physical therapy
Orthopaedic diseases and injuries
Office procedures and care of supplies and equipment
Operating room technique
Orientation to prosthetics and orthotics
Electives

Colorado Child Health Associate Bill*

CONCERNING THE PRACTICE AS A CHILD HEALTH ASSOCIATE, AND PROVIDING FOR THE REGULATION THEREOF

Be it enacted by the General Assembly of the State of Colorado:

Section 1. Short title. This act shall be known and may be cited as the "Child Health Associate Law."

Section 2. Definitions. (1) As used in this act:

(2) "Board" means the Colorado state board of medical examiners.

(3) "Pediatrics" means that branch of medicine which deals with the child and its growth and development and with the care, treatment, and prevention of diseases, injuries, and defects of children.

(4) "Physician" means a person who is licensed to practice medicine in this state.

(5) A "child health associate" is a person who, subject to the limitations provided by this act, practices pediatrics as an employee of and under the direction and supervision of a physician whose practice to a substantial extent is in pediatrics.

Section 3. Limitations on practice. (1) No person, other than a physician, shall practice as a child health associate in this state

---

*Enacted into law in 1969.

unless certified as such or as otherwise authorized pursuant to this act. Except as otherwise provided in this act, and except in the case of an emergency, a child health associate shall practice only in the professional office of the employing physician or physicians and only during the time when the employing physician or, in the case of a group of employing physicians, when one of such physicians whose practice to a substantial extent is in pediatrics, is directly and personally available. A child health associate may render pediatric services outside the professional office of the employing physician if such services either are rendered in the direct and personal presence of such physician, or consist of the follow-up care of a patient pursuant to the specific directions of such physician related to that particular patient.

(2) (a) A child health associate may prescribe drugs, except narcotic drugs, which have been approved by the board for prescription by child health associates. The board may approve drugs from the following categories for prescription by child health associates upon the recommendation of an advisory committee appointed by the board, consisting of a board member, a member of the department of pharmacology of the University of Colorado Medical Center, a practicing pediatrician, a licensed pharmacist, and a faculty member of the University of Colorado child health associate program:

(b) Proprietary and nonprescription drugs.

(c) (i) Specific drugs from the following categories of drugs for which a prescription is required:

    (ii) Immunologic agents
   (iii) Vitamins and dietary supplements
   (iv) Topical and oral decongestants
    (v) Oral laxatives and drugs affecting fecal consistency
   (vi) Oral or rectal antipyretics
  (vii) Oral nonnarcotic antitussives
 (viii) Oral expectorants
   (ix) Oral antihistaminics
    (x) Oral emetics in an emergency
   (xi) Local anti-infective agents
  (xii) Local antifungal agents
 (xiii) Local adrenal corticosteroids
 (xiv) Other agents for treatment of local skin conditions
  (xv) Oral or rectal antiemetics
 (xvi) Oral antidiarrheal agents
(xvii) Oral hematinic agents

(xviii) Injectible epinephrine, in an emergency
(xix) Diagnostic agents to determine the presence of various diseases
(xx) Antibiotics
(xxi) Chemotherapeutic agents

(3) Narcotic drugs may not be approved for prescription by child health associates.

(4) A child health associate shall not perform any operative or any cutting procedure or engage in the treatment of fractures, but this subsection (4) shall not be construed as prohibiting the rendering of such follow-up care as may be delegated by the employing physician.

(5) No more than one child health associate shall be employed at any one time by any one physician or, in the case of a group of employing physicians, no more than one child health associate shall be employed at any one time for each of such physicians whose practice to a substantial extent is in pediatrics.

(6) A child health associate shall practice in pediatrics only with respect to children who are the patients of the employing physician or physicians.

(7) (a) A child health associate may be employed only for work under the supervision of a physician who has been approved for such purpose by the board. The board shall approve any physician to employ child health associates if he furnishes evidence to the board that a substantial amount of his practice is concerned with pediatrics, that he is not then under investigation for unprofessional conduct as defined by law or that charges have not been filed because of such conduct, and that he is fully complying with all of the provisions of this act.

(b) Failure to continue compliance with the provisions of this subsection shall be grounds for withdrawal of such approval by the board.

(8) No child health associate shall use the title of doctor or associate with his name or any other term which would indicate to other persons that he is qualified to engage in the general practice of medicine.

Section 4. Responsibilities of physician. Nothing in this act shall be construed to relieve the physician of the professional or legal responsibility for the care and treatment of his patients. In furtherance of the purposes of this act, a physician utilizing the services of a child health associate pursuant to the provisions of this act shall not delegate to a child health associate the performance of, or permit a child health associate to perform, any act or duty not authorized by this act, and such physician shall exercise such direction, supervision, and control over such child health associate as will assure that patients under the care of such child health associate will receive medical care and treatment of high quality.

Section 5. Powers of board. The board shall have and exercise with respect to this act, all of the powers and duties granted it by article 1 of chapter 91, Colorado Revised Statutes 1963. It shall also have the power to make specific rules and regulations pertaining to the certification and regulation of child health associates.

Section 6. Qualifications—examination. (1) (a) The board shall certify as a child health associate and issue an appropriate certificate to any person who files a verified application therein upon a form prescribed by the board, tenders payment of the required fee, and furnishes evidence satisfactory to the board that the following qualifications have been met:

(b) Is at least twenty-one years of age;

(c) Is of good moral character;

(d) Is a citizen of the United States;

(e) Has completed a course of study approved by the board in an accredited college or university which includes the subjects of anatomy, physiology, biochemistry, pathology, pharmacology, microbiology, growth and development, child psychology and psychiatry, preventive pediatrics, and clinical pediatrics, and possesses at least a bachelor's degree from such college or university;

(f) Has completed an internship of at least one year approved by the board;

(g) Has passed an impartially administered examination given and graded by the board. Such examination may be in writing or oral, or both, and shall fairly test the applicant's knowledge in theoretical and applied pediatrics as it applies to the practice of a child health associate in at least the subjects of growth and development of the child, infant nutrition, immunization procedures, care of the normal newborn, and the common diseases of the child. The applicant's professional skill and judgment in the utilization of pediatric techniques and methods may also be examined.

Section 7. Certification by reciprocity. The board may certify as a child health associate in this state, without examination, a person who has been so certified or licensed by examination in another state of the United States which has requirements substantially equivalent to those in this act and who meets all requirements of section 6 of this act other than examination.

Section 8. Renewal. (1) Every person holding a certificate as a child health associate shall renew his certificate annually in the twelfth month following the date of issuance of his certificate.

(2) Any certificate not so renewed shall be suspended on the first day of the thirteenth month following the anniversary date of issuance of his certificate. A certificate so suspended may be reinstated during the following twelve months by payment of the renewal fee and a reinstatement fee as fixed by the board. Thereafter, a certificate so suspended may be reinstated only upon payment of all delinquent renewal fees and a reinstatement fee fixed by the board pursuant to section 11 of this act, following specific approval by the board.

(3) Renewal of a certificate shall be requested by every person certified as a child health associate upon a form which shall be furnished to him by the board during the tenth month of each year following the anniversary date of issuance of his certificate upon a form which shall be furnished to him by the board.

(4) A renewal request shall be accompanied by the prescribed fee together with evidence satisfactory to the board of the completion during the preceding twelve months of at least fourteen hours of postgraduate studies in pediatrics approved by the board.

Section 9. Denial, suspension, revocation, and probation. (1) (a) The board may deny an application for, suspend for a period not exceeding one year, revoke, or impose probationary conditions upon, a certificate for any of the following causes:

(b) A final conviction of a felony or any offense involving moral turpitude upon a plea or verdict of guilty or following a plea of nolo contendere;

(c) Use of drugs or intoxicating liquors to an extent which affects his professional competence;

(d) Obtaining or attempting to obtain a certificate by fraud or deception;

(e) Willfully violating any of the provisions of this act or any of the provisions of article 1 of chapter 91, C.R.S. 1963, as amended, which are applicable and which are not inconsistent with this act;

(f) Willfully and intentionally assisting in the practice or holding himself out to be a child health associate by one not certified under this article;

(g) Being legally determined to be mentally incompetent;

(h) Practicing as a child health associate other than as specified in sections 2 and 3 of this act;

(i) Being grossly negligent in the practice as a child health associate;

(j) Prescribing any drug which has not been approved for prescription by child health associates by the board;

Section 10. Disciplinary proceedings. Proceedings under this act shall be conducted in the manner specified by article 1 of chapter 91, and article 16 of chapter 3, C.R.S. 1963, as amended.

Section 11. Fees. (1) (a) The fees in connection with a certificate as a child health associate shall be as follows:

(b) For certificate by examination, not less than twenty-five dollars nor more than seventy-five dollars;

(c) For reexamination within one year, not less than fifteen dollars nor more than forty-five dollars;

(d) For certificate by reciprocity, not less than twenty-five dollars nor more than seventy-five dollars;

(e) For renewal of a certificate, not less than two dollars and fifty cents nor more than ten dollars;

(f) For reinstatement of a certificate, not less than five dollars nor more than twenty-five dollars;

(g) For reissuance of a lost or destroyed certificate, following approval of the board, ten dollars.

(2) Not later than the first day of June of each fiscal year, the board shall fix fees in each of the above categories within the stated limits in an amount which will produce sufficient revenue for the ensuing fiscal year not to exceed 120 percent of the anticipated expenses of the board for the operation of the child health associate program by the board for that year.

(3) All fees received by the board and all fines collected under the provisions of this act shall be paid to the department of revenue for transmission to the state treasurer who shall credit the same to the Colorado state board of medical examiners' fund.

(4) No fee shall be refunded.

Section 12. Violations and penalties. (1) Except as provided in section 13 of this act, it shall be unlawful for any person not certified under this act to practice as a child health associate or to hold himself out to be a child health associate in this state.

(2) Any person violating subsection (1) of this section, upon conviction, shall be punished by a fine of not less than twenty-five dollars nor more than three hundred dollars, or by imprisonment in the county jail for not more than ninety days, or by both such fine and imprisonment. Each violation shall be considered a separate offense.

Section 13. Exclusions. (1) (a) Nothing in this act shall be construed to limit:

(b) The activities and services of a child health associate student in pursuing an approved course of study or of an intern serving in an approved child health associate internship;

(c) The practice in this state for a period of not more than six months by a person certified as a child health associate in another state with requirements for such certification substantially equivalent to those in this act if such person first secures a permit from the board in a manner prescribed by the board, but the board may reduce such period to not less than thirty days;

(d) The employment of a child health associate by any federal, state, county, or municipal agency, but the child health associate so employed must be individually supervised by a designated and approved physician. Such physician shall supervise only one such child health associate. Such employment shall be subject to all the provisions of this act.

Section 14. Injunctive proceedings. (1) The board may, in the name of the people of the state of Colorado and through the attorney general of the state of Colorado, apply for an injunction in any court of competent jurisdiction to enjoin any person from committing any act prohibited by the provisions of this act.

(2) If it be established that any person has been or is committing an act prohibited by this act, the court or any judge thereof shall enter a decree perpetually enjoining said person from further committing such act.

(3) In case of violation of any injunction issued under the provision of this section, the court or any judge thereof may summarily try and punish the offender for contempt of court.

(4) Such injunctive proceedings shall be in addition to and not in lieu of all penalties and other remedies provided in this act.

Section 15. Feasibility study. During the eighth year after the effective date of this act, the board shall make a feasibility study and review of the provisions of this act to determine its effectiveness and accomplishments, and shall solicit the cooperation and advice of the Colorado medical society, the Colorado academy of general practice, the Colorado chapter of the American academy of pediatrics, the Rocky Mountain pediatric society, the Colorado osteopathic association, the faculty of the child health associate program of the University of Colorado medical center, and any such other interested person as the board or other named agencies may deem proper. The board shall report its findings and recommendations to the governor and the general assembly of the state of Colorado. Such report shall be issued subject to the provisions of Section 3-3-17, C.R.S. 1963, as amended.

Section 16. Effective date. This act shall take effect September 1, 1969.

Section 17. Safety clause. The general assembly hereby finds, determines, and declares that this act is necessary for the immediate preservation of the public peace, health, and safety.

Amendment to the New York Nursing Practice Act*

AN ACT TO AMEND THE EDUCATION LAW, IN RELATION TO THE PRACTICE OF NURSING

The People of the State of New York, represented in Senate and Assembly, do enact as follows:

Section 1. Sections sixty-nine hundred one through sixty-nine hundred seven of the education law are hereby renumbered to be sections sixty-nine hundred two through sixty-nine hundred eight, respectively.

§2. Such law is hereby amended by adding thereto a new section, to be section sixty-nine hundred one, to read as follows:

§6901. Definitions. As used in section sixty-nine hundred two:

1. "Diagnosing" in the context of nursing practice means that identification of and discrimination between physical and psychosocial signs and symptoms essential to effective execution and management of the nursing regimen. Such diagnostic privilege is distinct from a medical diagnosis.

2. "Treating" means selection and performance of those therapeutic measures essential to the effective execution and management of the nursing regimen, and execution of any prescribed medical regimen.

3. "Human Responses" means those signs, symptoms, and processes which denote the individual's interaction with an actual or potential health problem.

---

*Signed into law by Governor Rockefeller on March 15, 1972. The matter in *italics* is new; matter in brackets [ ] is old law to be omitted.

§3. Section sixty-nine hundred two of such law, as amended by chapter nine hundred ninety-four of the laws of nineteen hundred seventy-one, and as thus renumbered by section one of this act, is hereby amended to read as follows:

§6902. Definition of practice of nursing. 1. The practice of the profession of nursing as a registered professional nurse is defined as [performing service in the maintenance of health, prevention of illness, and care of the sick requiring the application of principles of nursing based on biological, physical, and social sciences such as supervising and providing nursing care and treatment through observation of a patient's condition, recording such observations, applying appropriate nursing measures, and executing orders concerning treatment and medication issued] *diagnosing and treating human responses to actual or potential health problems through such services as casefinding, health teaching, health counseling, and provision of care supportive to or restorative of life and well-being, and executing medical regimens prescribed* by a licensed or otherwise legally authorized physician or dentist. *A nursing regimen shall be consistent with and shall not vary any existing medical regimen.*

2. The practice of nursing as a licensed practical nurse is defined as performing [assigned duties and acts in the care of the sick under the direction of a registered professional nurse or a licensed or otherwise legally authorized physician or dentist requiring an understanding of nursing but not requiring the professional service as defined in subdivision one] *tasks and responsibilities within the framework of casefinding, health teaching, health counseling, and provision of supportive and restorative care under the direction of a registered professional nurse or licensed or otherwise legally authorized physician or dentist.*

§4. Section sixty-nine hundred eight of such law, as amended by chapter nine hundred ninety-four of the laws of nineteen hundred seventy-one, is hereby renumbered to be section sixty-nine hundred nine and is hereby amended to read as follows:

§6909. Special provision. *1.* Notwithstanding any inconsistent provision of any general, special, or local law, any licensed registered professional nurse or licensed practical nurse who voluntarily and without the expectation of monetary compensation renders first aid or emergency treatment at the scene of an accident or other emergency, outside a hospital, doctor's office, or any other place having proper and necessary medical equipment, to a person who is unconscious, ill, or injured shall not be liable for damages for injuries alleged to have been sustained by such person or for damages for the

death of such person alleged to have occurred by reason of an act or omission in the rendering of such first aid or emergency treatment unless it is established that such injuries were or such death was caused by gross negligence on the part of such registered professional nurse or licensed practical nurse. Nothing in this subdivision shall be deemed or construed to relieve a licensed registered professional nurse or licensed practical nurse from liability for damages for injuries or death caused by an act or omission on the part of such nurse while rendering professional services in the normal and ordinary course of her practice.

2. Nothing in this article shall be construed to confer the authority to practice medicine or dentistry.

§5. This act shall take effect immediately.

Chapter Five

Organizational Alternatives

Our analysis indicates that there is increasing role confusion among the various health professions, as well as a failure of organizational mechanisms and legal guidelines to provide an effective structure for health care delivery. More attention must focus on the way in which health professionals are organized to work together in giving health care.

As is apparent by its recurrence throughout the book, a most complex and crucial issue facing any emerging or expanding health profession is that of dependence versus independence of function. By function we mean those aspects of diagnosing, treating, operating, and prescribing which the physician may delegate. Fee for service and direct patient access are related problems which will be tied to the outcome of the dependence-independence issue.

In part, the dichotomy between dependence and independence can be resolved by *interdependence*, which promises to be a more productive framework from which to approach patient care. Interdependence evokes images of team planning and responsibility for the multifaceted and changing needs of the patient and his family. In some cases, the physician may relinquish his organizational jurisdiction over the patient's management, preferring instead to be a backup resource for the team's management of the patient. A model for team interdependence can be found in community mental health centers where responsibility for a given patient is shared by a team. The leader may not be a physician, but rather a nurse, psychologist, public health worker, or social worker. The success of interdependence in mental health care is a testimony to the feasibility of teamwork in health care.

CLOSING THE PROFESSIONAL GAP

We have borrowed from Dr. Edmund Pellegrino's writing about health team organization, finding his ideas both compelling and visionary.[1] He envisions the development of an array of transitory health teams who function together in the interests of patients. Teams are to be led in a fashion most appropriate to satisfying patient care needs at a given time. The captaincy of the team should be determined by the dominant features essential to the management of each patient.

The problems of leadership and coordination in implementing a well-formulated medical care plan are vital to successful teamwork. In addition to the skills already held by each professional, personal qualities of flexibility and a high level of trust are important. It may be difficult for some physicians to accept the idea of a shifting captaincy which truly shares responsibility and decision-making authority. The health team concept may be most fruitful with the PA filling the void of primary care created by the vanishing general practitioner. In primary care settings, the physician's assistant may assume a central patient care role with specialist physicians providing supervision and consultation.

ORGANIZATION OF THE HEALTH TEAM

The relationship of PAs to others on the health team will depend on their position in the numerous organizational arrangements open to them. Central to any health care worker's position on a table of organization are his functioning and accountability. These include supervision, categories of health care, health care settings, access to the patient, contractual arrangements, and compensation. These are not unique to the PA but pertain to every member of the health team.

Table 5-1 lists three basic types of organization to be considered in relating the PA to others on the health team: (1) vertical (figure 5-1), (2) horizontal (figure 5-2), and (3) circular (figure 5-3).

---

1. Edmund F. Pellegrino, "Closing the 'Profession Gap'—Some Notes on Unity of Purpose in the Health Professions." *In:* E. J. McTernan and R. O. Hawkins, editors, *Educating Personnel for the Allied Health Professions and Services: Administrative Considerations* (St. Louis: C. V. Mosby, 1972; Edmund F. Pellegrino, *The Changing Matrix of Clinical Decision-Making.* Ann Arbor, Michigan: University of Michigan Institute for Social Research, Survey Research Center (May 22, 1970), ch. IV, V.

Table 5–1. Organization of Health Care, Using Simplified Table-Of-Organization Models to Depict Dependent, Independent, Interdependent Functioning and Accountability

Table of Organization	*Functioning and Accountability*
I. Vertical or Hierarchical. Authoritarian	Dependent
II. Horizontal or Flattened. Egalitarian	Independent
III. Circular	Interdependent
(Figures 5–1, 5–2, 5–3, depict these arrangements.)	

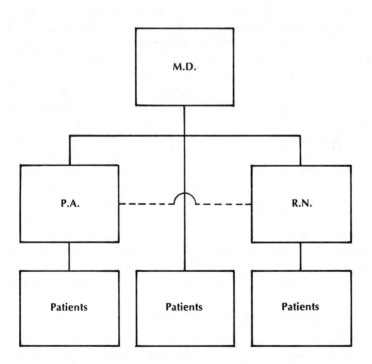

Figure 5–1. Vertical Table of Organization Showing Dependent Functioning and Accountability

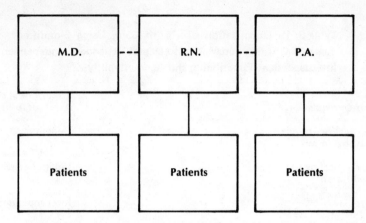

Figure 5–2. Horizontal Table of Organization Showing Independent Functioning and Accountability

A table of organization can only begin to suggest the myriad possibilities inherent in team care. The full implications of team care need to be pursued vigorously in search of empirical answers to the following concerns: What is the best composition for a given team to enable it to solve optimally the specific problems before it? What is the optimal assignment of tasks among existing health professionals and technicians? What new roles are required to carry out essential tasks now neglected? Who shall be the appropriate captain under varying conditions? How can there be input from all team members in ways that guarantee that input will be used constructively? What division of responsibility gives the team firm, clear direction and "keeps it from becoming a mob,"[2] or an endlessly indecisive committee?

The team approach to health care presents medical education with a new challenge. If the health team is to become a workable entity, its members must have some understanding of one another's competence, which means that they should receive part of their education together.[3] Trainees in health care professions especi-

---

2. Pellegrino, *The Changing Matrix of Clinical Decision-Making*, p. 22.

3. Evans lists the following problems which in his experience in Canada interfered with the coordination of education programs: (1) geographic isolation of classroom facilities for individual programs; (2) professional rivalry and the quest to retain a separate identity; (3) fear of domination by medicine; (4) dissimilarity of the knowledge base; and (5) different maturity levels of students. John R. Evans, "Coordination of Educational Programs" (Paper presented to the Second National Conference on Health Manpower, Ottawa, Canada, October 19–22, 1971), pp. 15–18.

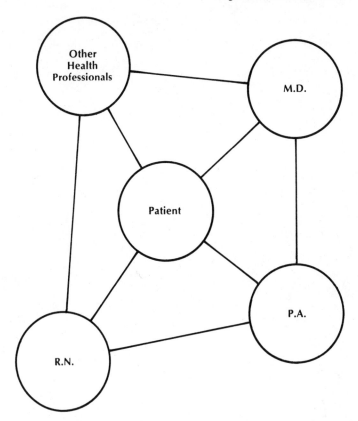

Figure 5–3. Circular Table of Organization Showing Interdependent Functioning and Accountability

ally need to share the clinical portion of their education. One way to do this is to organize students into health care teams so that they learn early in their professional life how to work interdependently for better patient care. Particularly in clinical education, student training groups comprised of future doctors, nurses, physician's assistants, and others need to be established. The goal in both the education and practice settings should be better patient care.

We have attempted to provide examples of basic practice arrangements available to the PA. An exhaustive analysis of organizational alternatives is beyond the scope of this book and the reader should consult the appropriate literature for a more comprehensive view.[4]

---

4. For a detailed bibliography, see Alvin H. Novack and Miriam Abramovitz, "Primary Care Health Teams: An Annotated Bibliography," prepared for the Maternal and Child Health Services, HSMHA, HEW (1973).

Chapter Six

Issues and Recommendations

PROBLEMS IN SEARCH OF RESOLUTION

We believe the physician's assistant concept holds great promise for improved health care. But like many innovations, the concept is not without problems. In the preceding pages we have endeavored to raise some of the important and often unexplored issues relating to the physician's assistant. Some of the most challenging issues have generated the questions below.

What does the future hold for physician's assistants? How can PAs be used most effectively where health needs are greatest? Will PAs be co-opted into specialty practice? How can PAs be located in areas of shortage with physician-nurse teams? Will flexible dependence to physicians be an effective legal framework for health care? Will PAs, like nurses, try to achieve independent status? How much and through what mechanism will PAs be paid?

Will the nursing profession try to insulate itself from this new development? How can the impending confrontation between the nurse and physician's assistant or their organizations be averted? What lessons about appropriate education and clinical training can be learned from nursing? What can be learned from the exodus of nurses from hospital practice? Can hospital conditions be improved to allow more effective utilization of nurses and other personnel?

How can PAs be deterred from following nurses and other professionals in seeking the status offered by higher educational credentials? What advanced entry to PA programs and what kinds of proficiency testing will increase the numbers of physician's assistants? Can a new midlevel patient care profession be made attractive equally to men and women?

143

Will medical schools support the needed experiments in health manpower education? What insights into improved preparation of physicians can PA programs offer medical schools? How might health professionals learn together in preparation for working together? How can the teaching of management skills be moved into medical education?

How might the scope of practice of physicians, nurses, physician's assistants, and other health workers be reexamined to reflect the realities of modern health care? How can new patient record systems be utilized to ensure quality patient care and encourage continuing education of health personnel? What will be the effect on the most important persons in the health care system—patients? Will they benefit by (1) improved care, (2) lower costs, (3) more personal service?

The recommendations that follow include proposals for addressing the major issues. We hope that all those concerned with improved health care will participate actively in the creative solution of these problems.

The following recommendations for action fall into two major categories: (1) immediate project support; and (2) in-depth policy studies, conferences, and polylogues. The first category contains proposals to be undertaken immediately by direct project support. The second category addresses issues that are better resolved by conferences and task force analyses, and of necessity require considerable additional planning.

These recommendations are based on the discussion in Chapters One through Five. A careful reading of these chapters is essential for full understanding of the recommendations. Textual references have been provided where appropriate.

RECOMMENDATIONS FOR IMMEDIATE PROJECT SUPPORT

1. *Physician's Assistant Program Support.* The Department of Health, Education and Welfare, the Veterans Administration, the armed services, and private foundations have all funded the training of physician's assistants.

a. The above groups should continue to maintain their leadership in improving the delivery of health care through support of especially innovative physician's assistant training programs.

b. Programs to train new health practitioners still should be viewed as experimental and as such deserve long range funding.

Such experiments are costly, but not unprecedented. For example, the Nurse Training Act awarded more than $700 million between 1965 and 1974 for scholarships, loans, and traineeships; construction and basic support for nursing education programs; and projects to improve nursing education and recruitment. In contrast, between 1972 and 1977, $65 million will have been awarded for new health practitioner programs (about one-half of which are nurse-based programs).

     c. Priority should be given to programs which train individuals broadly to give primary, preventive, and emergency care in a variety of settings (see p. 5).

     d. Priority should be given to programs which encompass the range of physician's assistant manpower sources available including: individuals with extensive experience and little formal education, e.g., military corpsmen; science-major college graduates with little health experience; and health professionals who desire an extended or expanded role, e.g., inhalation therapists and pharmacists (see pp. 5–6).

     e. Priority should be given to programs which offer admission without regard to sex or race (see pp. 15–16).

     f. Priority should not be given to training programs utilizing rigid education requirements or other arbitrary admissions criteria (see pp. 7–11 and Chapter Three).

     g. Priority should be given to programs that can develop appropriate academic credit for their graduates.

     2. *Maldistribution of Health Services.* Maldistribution of services is one of the major problems in health care delivery today. If the physician's assistant movement fails to address itself to maldistribution, its impact will be significantly lessened. In light of the current financing mechanisms for health care, we believe there will be strong incentives for graduates of physician's assistant programs (even in primary care) to practice in fields and locations where the remuneration is greatest, namely specialties in suburban and urban centers (see pp. 11–14). A variety of economic incentives could be developed to ameliorate this situation.

     Experience with recent medical school graduates suggests that multimedia communication links between geographically remote practice settings and university medical centers can equal financial inducements. In addition, the potential of the problem-oriented medical record for self-assessment may provide an important reinforcement for individuals working in isolated areas, far removed from peer review and the advantages of daily interchange with colleagues.

a. We therefore recommend support of demonstration projects utilizing various economic, communications, and other mechanisms to encourage the location of physician's assistants in areas of medical shortage. Stipends and income assurance subsidies are two possible financial approaches. These projects should take cognizance of the success and failures of earlier attempts, such as loan forgiveness.

b. The development of cost-effective communications links between geographically remote practice settings and university medical centers should be supported.

c. We recommend implementation and promotion of the problem-oriented medical record as a uniform tool for self-assessment and evaluation.

d. Because physician's assistants will be largely dependent on physicians and will function in teams with physicians, **we recommend support of demonstration projects that locate health teams (including physicians, nurses, and physician's assistants) in areas of need to deliver health care.**

3. *Advanced Entry to Physician's Assistant Programs.*
Early evidence from the first physician's assistant programs supports the widely held belief that large numbers of individuals currently employed in health occupations are eager to expand their role and would like to deliver primary care as physician's assistants (see pp. 5–6). Physician's assistant programs should be "modified" in length and content to account for the previous health experience and expertise of the applicant, e.g., nursing, pharmacy, physical therapy. The following recommendations focus particularly on nurses because they comprise by far the largest health manpower resource.

a. We recommend support for existing or proposed physician's assistant programs that make special provision for advanced entry for other health professionals.

b. Priority should be given to diploma nurses whose opportunities for expanded functioning are especially limited by our current degree-oriented health care system (see pp. 46–49). We do not believe this recommendation is subject to the "rob Pauline to pay Peter" argument frequently used against physician's assistant programs that accept nurses. Modified physician's assistant programs are not likely to lure contented nurses or those baccalaureate nurses who can find an expanded role through "nurse practitioner" or master's degree nursing programs.

We believe that a modified physician's assistant approach

will be attractive to some of the 650,000 registered nurses prematurely "in retirement" who would welcome the opportunity to work in a health profession outside of "nursing."

c. Support should be given to pilot programs which meld nurse clinician preparation and the physician's associate (Type A) education into a single middle level health care profession under the auspices of medical schools or health sciences divisions of universities. Thorough evaluation of such experimental programs will be essential.

d. The development and testing of proficiency and equivalency measurements should be undertaken to facilitate advanced entry.

4. *Proficiency Measurements for the Physician's Assistant.* The development of adequate proficiency tests to measure the competence of physician's assistants is vitally important to the innovative and flexible development of the PA concept. To be effective, such tests must be designed to reflect competence in practice settings as well as basic knowledge. We applaud the leadership taken by the National Board of Medical Examiners and the American Medical Association in beginning development of such tests.

a. We therefore recommend that appropriate support be made available to the development of proficiency examinations for physician's assistants (of both the generalist and specialist types) so that this important effort can be facilitated (see pp. 91–92).

b. It is essential that the tests be available to health workers possessing a broad range of experience in patient care and not be limited only to graduates of accredited physician's assistant training programs.

5. *Common Teaching in the Health Professions.* As the number and variety of physician's assistants expand, expensive duplication of teaching and curricula will continue unless proper coordination is achieved. We believe common teaching is essential. Health professionals at all levels who must work together on behalf of patient care should be able to learn together.

a. Support should be given to demonstration projects to develop and test common teaching within and between institutions for the training of a broad variety of health workers. Provision should be made for appropriate modification of common teaching following testing.

b. Efforts should be made to identify the core knowledge that is required for all midlevel health workers in the delivery of primary care.

c. Demonstration projects should be undertaken in medical schools to offer a course such as Anatomy and Physiology, which is common to all health profession students, in discrete credit units of progressive difficulty which provide entry, exit, and reentry points for all levels of health professionals.

d. Research should be undertaken with clear regard to the kinds of clinical tasks which health workers will perform and should not be constrained by traditional educational requirements.

6. *Management Skills and Health Teams.* As the knowledge base in health care continues to expand and as specialties increase, much of health care will be delivered by teams of health professionals. In light of this, the physician will become a manager and supervisor of health care delivery in many settings and will need to learn how to delegate and apportion tasks in the most effective fashion (see Chapter Five, "Organizational Alternatives").

a. We therefore recommend the support of courses, as part of the medical school curriculum, which analyze the roles of physicians in team health care delivery and provide management skills to physicians.

b. The physician will not always be the captain or primary manager of these teams. We therefore recommend that courses in other health programs (e.g., nursing and physician's assistant) be established to provide necessary organization management skills. Courses already being given in management skills in business and other schools may provide excellent models.

c. Such courses should be linked to practice systems using the health team concept, and these systems should be evaluated for their effectiveness in teaching the practice of medicine as well as improving the standard of care.

7. *Comparative Study of Levels of Nursing Education.* With the objective of obtaining an estimate of the potential performance levels of various categories of PAs, a comparative study should be undertaken of the patient care performance of nurses trained at the associate degree, diploma, and baccalaureate levels. Ten years have passed since the ANA position paper recommended the phasing out of hospital schools of nursing. Adequate data should be available now to evaluate the effect on the quality of care of baccalaureate and associate degree nursing education compared to diploma nursing education. As yet, no such *adequate* study has been undertaken.

a. An indepth analysis and evaluation of the comparative effectiveness of baccalaureate, associate degree, and diploma nurses in providing quality health care should be undertaken immediately.

The results of such a comparison would inform the current development of various levels of physician's assistant programs. Especially needed is the identification of the most effective mix of didactic and clinical components of an educational program for health care. A good comparative study of nursing also would provide a model for the evaluation of varying educational levels in other health professions.

b. The comparative study should seek neither to reverse nor to support the ANA decision to phase out diploma schools, but to quantify and identify the best that each type of nurse preparation brings to patient care. The resultant mutual respect and subsequent interchange of ideas among the different types of programs should contribute to much needed unification of the fragments that make up the nursing profession.

c. A research institution, without a vested interest in the outcome, should conduct the comparative study.

INDEPTH POLICY STUDIES, CONFERENCES, AND POLYLOGUES

We believe that much is wrong with the way health manpower problems are often discussed and analyzed. The organized health professions have not provided needed leadership. Too frequently their attempts have floundered in a bog of concerns over professionalism, authority, and status. Too frequently the majority of representatives are elder statesmen in the health field who do not have to live with the solutions they propose. Meanwhile, the consumer insists on a greater voice in the delivery of medical care.

Any effort to assign the appropriate place of the physician's assistant must take full cognizance of the dynamic and vastly accelerating needs for medical care which will be delivered increasingly by interdisciplinary teams working in a variety of settings (see pp. 137–141).

As stated earlier, the problems posed by the physician's assistant often are not unique to the PA, but in fact are part of the critical issues affecting our health care system today (see pp. 1–6). To explore these many complex issues requires that members of the health professions, hospital administration, law, community and regional health planning, business, and the public be brought together in the most productive interdisciplinary endeavors. For most effective results, this interplay should occur at three levels.

1. *In-depth Policy Studies.* **An extensive and continuing analysis of issues should be undertaken under prestigious and neutral sponsorship.** Multidisciplinary task forces should be formed to focus on such issues as: (1) appropriate levels, ratings, and nomenclature of midlevel health workers (see p. 11); (2) alternative economic reimbursement mechanisms (see p. 17); (3) definitions of scope of practice of the physician's assistant, the physician, the nurse, and other health professionals (see pp. 99–104); (4) procedures for improving equity of access to health care (see pp. 11–14); (5) accountability through licensure, certification, accreditation, and other mechanisms (see pp. 88–106); (6) the development of alternative team arrangements for health care (see pp. 137–141); (7) amelioration of competition and friction among existing and developing health professions (see pp. 49–56); and (8) the utilization of proficiency and equivalency measures for health workers (see pp. 88–93).

We envision a major study of the Carnegie or Rockefeller Commission type. Commission representation should be diverse and comprehensive. The foundations have a key role here and could provide the ideal mechanism for this study. Such a major research effort would most likely require 24 months for the completion of analysis and publication of findings. Adequate communication and cooperation with the appropriate federal agencies and the newly developed Institute of Medicine of the National Academy of Sciences would be desirable. Improved patient care should remain the paramount concern throughout.

2. *Conferences.* **A series of major conferences should be held to provide a forum at which to frame important issues.** Appropriate issues are those mentioned for analysis in the preceding paragraph. A Macy Conference format could be extremely effective.[1]

A follow-up Macy Conference could provide the participants an opportunity to reflect upon the continuing evolution of the issues and to evaluate the progress of steps recommended at the first conference.

---

1. A highly successful Macy Conference was held in November 1972 and its proceedings were published and distributed widely. V. Lippard and E. Purcell, eds, *Intermediate-Level Health Practitioners*, (New York: Josiah Macy Jr. Foundation, 1973).

3. *Polylogues.* We suggest a series of polylogues. By this we envision a series of informal two or three day retreats in which representatives of the health care professions and other disciplines are able to discuss freely the promises and problems posed by the physician's assistant. It is imperative that the individuals involved be able to discard their organization mantles and thus be free to converse with candor.

The purpose of this approach is to give controversial viewpoints that otherwise might not find the light of day an opportunity to be expressed, and to influence the thinking of others in health care leadership. Polylogue participants should be asked to decide how best to convey their ideas and recommendations for use by the larger study commission (see p. 150).

Participants from both within and without the health care professions should be sought who are likely to provide fresh insights and new perspectives. We fully expect that some of the most sage thinking will come from what seem to be unlikely sources.

Chapter Seven

Epilogue: New Health Practitioners in Evolution

This chapter presents in capsule form an update of a number of important events which have occurred during the past three years.

The epilogue will also elaborate on the theme[1] of the new health practitioner as a major experiment in social change. We believe that new health practitioners are of revolutionary importance and represent the human equivalent of a major new health technology whose impact is potentially comparable to the development of the antibiotics or new vaccines.

CURRENT STATUS OF THE PA MOVEMENT

Physician's assistants comprise a significant portion of the new health practitioner profession. The current status of the PA movement, not including nurse practioners,[2] follows:

Programs

- The physician's assistant is now a well-established health occupation with 48 AMA accredited training programs throughout the country (see Appendix A).

Graduates

- With more than 1,000 now being produced annually, the number of PA graduates is expected to reach 3,000 by September 1975.

---

1. This theme was underscored in the Authors' Note to the Second Edition (see pp. xvii–xviii).
2. Nurse practitioners will be discussed later in the epilogue.

153

Thus, PAs are beginning to make a quantitative impact on the nation's health manpower.

Male and Female

- Originally, the PA was an ex-military corps*man*. Today the ratio of male to female PA graduates is 7:3.
- Women entering the field are expected to increase to at least 40 percent.

Utilization and Deployment

- Nearly 80 percent of graduate PAs work in primary care settings.
- One-third of graduate PAs work in settings serving populations of 10,000 or less.
- Nearly half of all graduates work in settings serving populations of 20,000 or less.
- The American Hospital Association has actively promoted the use of PAs as a means of extending medical services in hospitals.[3]
- In some institutions, PAs are replacing medical house staff. This trend may accelerate if the pipeline of foreign medical graduates into the U.S. is closed, as advocated by many.

Reimbursement

- The Social Security Administration has undertaken a two year experiment in medicare reimbursement for "physician extenders"—PAs and nurse practitioners. Under the experiment, approximately 1000 practice settings will receive reimbursement at physician rates for specific delegated medical tasks performed by physician extenders.

Professional Organization

- The American Academy of Physicians' Assistants and The Association of Physician Assistant Programs opened a national executive office in Washington, D.C. in the summer of 1974 to provide information and coordinate Academy and Association activities.
- *The P.A. Journal—A Journal for New Health Practitioners* (originally called *The Physician's Associate*) is the official publication of the American Academy of Physicians' Assistants. Established in 1971, the journal has attempted to foster communication and collegiality among a variety of new health practitioners.
- Three annual national New Health Practitioner Conferences have

---

3. American Hospital Association, "Statement on the Role of the Physician's Assistant in the Hospital" (approved by the Council on Professional Services, March 8, 1974). (See pp. 167–171).

been well attended and have addressed the latest developments in the profession.

NURSING REVISITED

The physician's assistant movement has served as an added impetus to excellence in clinical nursing.[4] The proliferation of programs to prepare nurse practitioners is partly attributable to the physician's assistant movement.

Programs

- As of 1975, nearly 150 programs offer registered nurses formal didactic and clinical preparation for an expanded role in general primary care (see Appendix A).
- Nearly 100 programs award a nurse practitioner certificate.
- Fifty-four universities and colleges offer a masters degree to prepare clinical nurse specialists.

Graduates

- To date, there are approximately 4,000 graduates of nurse practitioner programs.
- Another 2,000 are currently enrolled in nurse practitioner and masters degree clinical nurse specialist programs.
- The majority of masters degree graduates are engaged in teaching, administration, or research and thus are able to provide only a minimum of direct patient services.

Reimbursement

- Nursing is seeking direct reimbursement for independent nursing services under medicaid and medicare. Among efforts toward this purpose is Senate Bill S104 introduced by Senator Daniel Inouye in January 1975.

Professional Organization

- The ANA has defined for purposes of clarification the terms *Nurse Practitioner, Nurse Clinician,* and *Clinical Nurse Specialist* (see pp. 173–174).
- Organized nursing continues its advocacy of academic credentials as a requisite to professionalism. The New York State Nurses' Association "Resolution 1985" recommends that by 1985 the minimum requirement to be a registered nurse is the baccalau-

---

4. Alex Kacen, "The Physician Assistant: An Added Impetus to Excellence in Nursing," *The Physician's Associate* 3, no. 1 (January 1973):9–13.

reate degree. Theoretically, anyone without the BSN would not be an RN and presumably would be designated an LPN. The implications of closing the diploma and associate degree routes to the RN are as yet unclear.

PROGRESS IN THE LAW AND PROFESSIONAL STANDARDS

The new health practitioner effort over the past three years has seen continued progress concerning licensure at the state level, and certification and accreditation at the national level.

PA Legislation

- Enabling legislation for PAs has been passed in 37 states. There are two basic types of legislation which cover PAs—delegation and regulation (see Appendix B).
- The National Board of Medical Examiners designed the National Certification Examination for the Assistant to the Primary Care Physician, offered for the first time in December of 1973. Despite efforts to discourage nurses from taking the exam as not being in their best interest (see pp. 175–176), 10 percent of the examinees in 1973 were nurse practitioners. Results of the first two exams showed that PAs and nurse practitioners fared comparably.
- In unprecedented collaboration, 14 national health professional organizations convened the National Commission on Certification of Physician's Assistants in August 1974. The commission has established eligibility and passing levels for the National Board of Medical Examiners' Certification Examination.

Accreditation of PA Programs

- As of May 1975, 48 programs had been accredited by the AMA and its joint review committee, which includes the American Academy of Family Physicians, the American Academy of Pediatrics, the American Academy of Physician's Assistants, the American College of Physicians, and the American Society of Internal Medicine.

Nurse Practice Act Legislation

- During the past three years, a majority of states have reexamined their antiquated nurse practice acts and some states have amended them. These amendments have taken several forms, notably the New York State Nurses' Association's revision (see pp.

106–110 and pp. 133–135). More promising for nurse practitioners are those amendments that promote cooperation between medicine and nursing through mechanisms of joint regulation.

Nurse Practitioner Certification

• The ANA has undertaken a certification process for nurse practitioners. In contrast to certification of the PA as a generalist, ANA certification is by specialty including: community health, geriatrics, maternal/child, medical/surgical, and psychiatric and mental health.

Accreditation of Nurse Programs

• The ANA and NLN are developing an accreditation process jointly for nurse practitioner certificate programs.
• The NLN remains the accrediting body for masters degree programs preparing clinical nurse specialists.

Malpractice

• Although malpractice is one of the gravest concerns facing all physicians, the utilization of increasing numbers of new health practitioners has not resulted in a rash of law suits, as some had feared (see pp. 87–88).

INTERDEPENDENCE

Medicine and nursing are increasingly realizing that health care can be improved through collaboration between the two professions.

Collaboration in Practice

• One mode of interdependence is joint physician-nurse practice. Literature on the use of nurse practitioners has come primarily from medical and nursing academic centers—not from the practices themselves. One effort to remedy this lack of information is the current preparation by the National Joint Practice Commission of a casebook of 22 sample physician-nurse joint practices. The casebook is designed to promote replication of joint practice.

Collaboration in Education

• Another mode of interdependence is the joint training of physicians and nurses which is being demonstrated successfully at institutions such as the University of Rochester and the University of California at Davis.

- Joint education of physicians, nurse practitioners, and PAs is underway at the Medical College of Georgia in Augusta and at the Indiana University School of Medicine in Indianapolis.

Professional Collaboration Falters

- In contrast to these encouraging developments, a new schism arose between the ANA and the American Academy of Pediatrics as to which organization should have certification responsibility for pediatric nurse practitioners. This dispute resulted in the defection of many pediatric nurse practitioners to the National Association of Pediatric Nurse Associates and Practitioners (NAP–NAP).

Policy Studies

- As proposed in the recommendations of the first edition, a Macy Conference on "Intermediate-Level Health Practitioners" was held in 1972 to address many of the policy issues confronting the field.[5]
- A 24 month Institute of Medicine Study begun in Spring 1975 is examining the functions of all health practitioners in primary care.
- A report on federally funded "physician extender" programs and related issues was prepared for Congress by the General Accounting Office in April 1975 and contains important recommendations for further HEW action.[6]

WHO'S AILING AND WHAT DO THEY NEED?

In light of these developments, consider the following facts:
Out of a typical sample of 1000 adults in America, in any one month 750 will experience some form of illness or injury. Of these, only about one-third, or 250, consult a physician. Of these, nine are hospitalized and five are sent to a second physician for consultation or therapy. Only one out of the 750 is referred to a university medical center. Thus, the patients coming to the community physician are very different from those who reach the university medical center, the latter usually having been filtered twice before admission.[7]

---

5. Vernon W. Lippard and Elizabeth F. Purcell eds., *Intermediate-Level Health Practitioners*, (New York: Josiah Macy Jr. Foundation, 1973).

6. U.S. General Accounting Office (Report to the Congress of the United States), "Progress and Problems in Training and Use of Assistants to Primary Care Physicians," no. MWD–75–35 (April 8, 1975).

7. Kerr L. White, T. Franklin Williams and Bernard G. Greenberg, "The Ecology of Medical Care," *New England Journal of Medicine* 265, no. 19 (November 2, 1961):885–892.

An indication of the important medical problems facing the primary care physician can be obtained by examining the leading causes of death in America today. Most of these conditions are chronic progressive diseases for which there is presently no known cure. Included are heart disease, cancer, cerebrovascular disease, diabetes, cirrhosis, arteriosclerosis, bronchitis, and emphysema (see Table 7-1). The principal interventions for these problems, once diagnosed, involve the maintenance of a lifelong treatment plan and in some cases a modification of behavior, such as weight loss for the obese and reduction of smoking for those with heart or chronic lung disease. Most of this maintenance can be performed by new health practitioners.

Another major killer today is accidental death, which ranks fourth overall and is the leading cause of death between the ages of one and 44. Yet treatment of life-threatening accidents fall largely outside the realm of the primary care physician in the community. Lifesaving measures for accidents depend principally on rapid emergency medical response by appropriately trained emergency medical technicians who have the necessary equipment and expertise to treat at the scene and transport a patient quickly and effectively to a hospital's emergency department where more definitive therapy can occur.

An even more important perspective on the patient coming to the practicing physician in the community can be obtained by looking at the most common problems he sees. The following conditions are listed in descending order of frequency and are based on a two year study of family practice in Monroe County, New York during the years 1971 to 1973.[8] The figure next to each condition is the number of thousands of cases seen during the study period:

1. Upper respiratory infections—2.8
2. Pharyngitis or sore throats—2.7
3. Lacerations, sprains, abrasions—2.5
4. Otitis media (the common middle ear infection in children)—1.7
5. Obesity—1.6
6. Hypertension—1.4
7. Anxiety states—1.3
8. Bronchitis—1.1
9. Vaginitis, cervicitis, and other female infections—1.0
10. Depression—0.7

---

8. Collin Baker, "What's Different About Family Medicine?" *Journal of Medical Education* 49, no. 3 (March 1974):229–235.

Table 7–1.   The Ten Leading Causes of Death in 1900 and 1971

Cause of Death (1900)	Deaths per 100,000 persons	Percent of all deaths	Cause of Death (1971)	Deaths per 100,000 persons	Percent of all deaths
All causes	1,719.1	100.0	All causes	929.0	100.0
Influenza and pneumonia	202.2	11.8	Diseases of the heart	358.4	38.6
Tuberculosis (all forms)	194.4	11.3	Malignant neoplasms	160.9	17.3
Gastritis, etc.	142.7	8.3	Cerebrovascular diseases	100.6	10.8
Diseases of the heart	137.4	8.0	Accidents	53.8	5.8
Vascular lesions affecting central nervous system	106.9	6.2	Influenza and pneumonia	27.2	2.9
Chronic nephritis	81.0	4.7	Certain diseases of early infancy	19.2	2.1
All accidents	72.3	4.2	Diabetes mellitus	18.2	2.0
Malignant neoplasms (cancer)	64.0	3.7	Cirrhosis of liver	15.5	1.7
Certain diseases of early infancy	62.6	3.6	Arteriosclerosis	15.5	1.7
Diphtheria	40.3	2.3	Bronchitis, emphysema, and asthma	14.5	1.6
			All other causes	145.3	15.6

Source: *Progress in Health Services*, vol. 10, no. 2, February 1961. *Monthly Vital Statistics Report, Annual Summary for the United States, 1971.* U.S. Department of Health, Education, and Welfare, National Center for Health Statistics, Aug. 30, 1972.

The next five are diabetes; low back problems; urinary tract infections; sinusitis; and warts, nevi, and other skin lesions.

This list makes up what is often called by academicians the worried well and the walking wounded, but it is the bread and butter of general medical practice. The emphasis in medical education is not on these problems and their management but on the unusual, the esoteric interesting case known as the "fascinoma" in medical school jargon. How can a physician be educated to face the problems of the community if he sees only 13-hundredths of 1 percent of sick adults in society and four-tenths of 1 percent of patients who consult a physician? This is the population which is referred to university medical centers where young physicians are educated. They and other students of the health professions receive an unrealistic impression of medicine's role in contemporary Western society.[9]

Some medical schools would argue that they are exempt from this indictment, insisting that other schools should be responsible for training primary care physicians so that they can prepare researchers, teachers, and subspecialists for academic medicine. Yet no more than 15 percent of any medical school's graduates enter academic careers. What about the other 85 percent in even those schools? They clearly do not receive the training they need. This phenomenon has been called "educational malpractice" by two noted commentators on the academic medical scene.[10]

FIT, NONFIT, AND UNFIT

What are the reasons for the lack of fit between what is taught in medical schools and what is needed by physicians in medical practice? Two major factors are subspecialization and the enormous success of biomedical research.

First consider the issue of specialization. From Kerr White's data, it is reasonable to postulate that our medical schools should train many more generalists capable of dealing with a broad range of community health problems. It appears that a much smaller number of specialists and subspecialists are needed to handle the small percentage of patients who require their care. If one looks at the ratio of generalists to specialists in England, there seems to be a good fit between what is needed and what is produced. There are 22,000 generalists and 8,000 specialists there. In the United States,

---

9. White et al, p. 890.

10. Joel J. Alpert and Evan Charney, *The Education of Physicians for Primary Care* (Washington, D.C.: USDHEW Pub. no. [HRA] 74–3113, Autumn 1973).

on the other hand, we have 70,000 generalists and 280,000 specialists.[11] Clearly things are topsy-turvy here. The reasons for the malignant growth of specialization in the U.S. and the decline of the family physician have been discussed in many writings and will not be reviewed here.[12] It is clear that specialization has helped cause the lack of fit between what is produced by our medical schools and what is needed by our people.

The enormous growth of biomedical research in the 1950s and 1960s, largely underwritten by taxpayer's dollars through the National Institutes of Health, helped us eradicate many of our acute medical problems. New vaccines, drugs, and surgical procedures have had substantial impact on major causes of death and disability. But an unwanted side effect of this success has been an overemphasis on the technological, the scientific, and the measurable—at the expense of the intuitive, the caring, and the human. The results are legions of specialty physicians who, while technically competent to handle a limited range of diseases, are often not competent to manage a broad range of medical problems, not to mention the related psychosocial concomitants to these problems. A new interest in humanism in medicine is one response to this situation.[13] This has clear implications for the new health practitioner who is being trained in many programs to address these problems.

Some critics of our increasingly technological, specialized, and dehumanized medicine foresee the end of medicine as we now know it. Ivan Illich, the well-known critic of the educational establishment, has charged the medical establishment with causing many of society's ills in addition to being unresponsive to others.[14] Rick J. Carlson expresses similar sentiments in his book entitled *The End of Medicine*.[15]

---

11. Paul B. Beeson, "Some Good Features of the British National Health Service," *Journal of Medical Education* 49, no. 1 (January 1974):43–49.

12. Michael Crichton, *Five Patients* (New York: Bantom Books, 1970), p. 209; Robert H. Ebert, "The Medical School," *Scientific American* 229, no. 3 (September 1973):139–148; Victor R. Fuchs, *Who Shall Live—Health, Economics and Social Choice* (New York: Basic Books, 1974), p. 168; David E. Rogers, "The Unity of Health: Reasonable Quest or Impossible Dream?" *Journal of Medical Education* 46 no. 12 (December 1971):1047–1056.

13. Mary M. Belknap, Robert A. Blau and Rosalind N. Grossman, *Case Studies and Methods in Humanistic Medical Care* (San Francisco: Institute for the Study of Humanistic Medicine, 1975), p. 110; Naomi Remen, *The Masculine Principle, The Feminine Principle and Humanistic Medicine* (San Francisco: Institute for the Study of Humanistic Medicine, 1975), p. 105.

14. Ivan Illich, *Medical Nemesis* (London: Calder and Boyars, 1974).

15. Rick J. Carlson, *The End of Medicine* (New York: John Wiley & Sons, Inc., 1975).

Although we hardly foresee the "end of medicine," as the costs of care go out of sight, physicians become less and less accessible, and the treatment experience becomes less human, we believe that more people will ask, if not demand, that the lack of fit we have described be redressed. There are several solutions to the lack of fit. We contend that most of these solutions can and must come from within our health care system.

First, more generalist physicians and fewer specialists must be produced. This means an increase in the number of primary care doctors, including family practitioners, general internists, and general pediatricians. To do so will require a reduction of residency positions in some specialties while increasing substantially the number of general physician residency slots.

Second, we must modify the education of all physicians to include a better understanding of the intuitive and caring functions which physicians should perform.[16] Michael Halberstam cites alienation as the most common illness of Western man. Surely our health care system shouldn't contribute to this alienation. We must bring common sense back into our health care and, to quote Halberstam: "help the obese patient lose weight, the smoker to abandon cigarettes and the heavy drinker to cut down or cut out alcohol."[17] The primary care physician must be trained to handle these problems, or at least manage others who are. Other solutions are discussed by Walsh McDermott in his paper on general medical care.[18] Many of these deserve serious consideration, but they will not be reviewed here.

THE HUMAN EQUIVALENT OF A NEW TECHNOLOGY

When discussing change in social systems, our colleague Dr. McDermott has made a very telling point. He points out that major social change usually follows major technological change and without major new technology we are much less likely to see major social change. There are many examples of this—from the wheel and inclined plane; to the discovery of moveable type; to the telephone and

---

16. Robert E. Ornstein, *The Psychology of Consciousness* (San Francisco: W. H. Freeman and Company, 1972), p. 247.

17. Michael J. Halberstam, "Liberal Thought, Radical Theory and Medical Practice," *New England Journal of Medicine* 284, no. 21 (May 27, 1971):1180–1185.

18. Walsh McDermott, "General Medical Care—Identification and Analysis of Alternative Approaches," *Johns Hopkins Medical Journal* 135, no. 5 (November 1974):292–321.

the airplane. In medicine, the discovery of anesthesia and the antibiotics are classic examples of technology that makes a difference. The development of antituberculous drugs has wiped out the need for the great number of tuberculosis sanitoriums (see Table 7-1). Similarly, polio vaccine has cut deeply into the need for iron lungs and wheel chairs.

One might legitimately ask, Is there a new technology which could be applied to the problems of general medical care, that might help solve our problems of lack of fit between the products of our medical schools and the needs of our society? What technology can help to solve the need to manage many common medical illnesses and do so in a human, caring fashion? *We submit that there is none.* There are technological adjuncts to be sure—the computer to maintain records efficiently and aid in some diagnosis; the autoanalyzer, which can do 12 laboratory studies in less time and at less cost than older methods; and television, which can aid some kinds of medical consultation. But there will never be a substitute for a health professional who can provide what Dr. McDermott calls "science-based samaritanism," defined as the ability to support and help the unwell based on a knowledge of science.[19]

Although we submit that no new technology will ever provide science-based samaritanism, we suggest that the human equivalent of a new technology already exists which can provide it. We are referring to the variety of new health practitioners on the American health scene. In contrast to traditional health practitioners, such as the physician, the new health practitioner is trained to recognize and manage the common health problems which face us all. And all of the strong NHP programs provide a solid base in clinical science as well. New health practitioners bring several important advantages that no technology, or other human equivalent that we know of, can match.

First, recent data indicates that greater than 77 percent of graduates are working in general primary care. They are filling the role intended.[20]

Second, the cost of NHP production is about one-sixth that of physician production. Most training programs are two years in length in contrast to the six to eight years postcollege training needed to produce a primary care physician and the cost per year is approximately one-half of the annual cost of producing a fully trained physician.

---

19. Ibid., p. 293.
20. Donald W. Fisher, "Physician Assistant—A Profile of the Profession" (Presented at the 3rd Annual Conference on New Health Practitioners, St. Louis, April 7, 1975).

Third, under prepayment systems the cost of medical care should go down or at least the rate of increase will be reduced. NHPs average $14,000–$15,000 in annual salary as compared to $30,000 to $40,000 for a general physician.

Fourth, all patient acceptance studies are favorable at greater than 90 percent. This is certainly as good as physician acceptance, not to mention acceptance rates of new technologies in general.[21]

Fifth, quality of care studies indicate that for the job defined, NHPs do a job that is equal in quality to that of the physician.[22] Care is often more satisfying to a patient because the NHP has more time to spend on education, counseling, and guidance.

It is too early to determine the impact of NHPs on geographic distribution of health care services, but we believe that they will have salutory, if limited, effect by helping to keep physicians in underserved areas. Fundamentally, they can help to enhance the quality of life of the personal encounter physician who works in underserved areas.

Of course a number of problems remain, many of which have been addressed in the preceding chapters. But in our view, few developments on the modern health care scene offer as much hope for reestablishing the kind of fit in health care that people in our society so desperately want. And in our view, the proper training and utilization of new health practitioners should go a long way toward helping the health professions fulfill their commitment to the society they serve.

---

21. Richard A. Henry, "Use of Physician's Assistants in Gilchrist County, Florida," *Health Services Reports* 87, no. 8 (October 1972):687–692; Eva D. Cohen, *An Evaluation of Policy Related Research and Expanded Roles of Health Workers: Executive Summary* (New Haven: Yale University School of Medicine, Office of Regional Activities and Continuing Education, October 1974).

22. Fernando J. deCastro and Ursula T. Rolfe, "An Evaluation of New Primary Pediatric Paraprofessionals," *Journal of Medical Education* 49, no. 2 (February 1974):192–193; Louis L. Fine and Henry K. Silver, "Comparative Diagnostic Abilities of Child Health Associate Interns and Practicing Pediatricians," *The Journal of Pediatrics* 83, no. 2 (August 1973):332–335; Pavel Machotka, John E. Ott, John B. Moon and Henry K. Silver, "Competence of Child Health Associates I. Comparison of their Basic Science and Clinical Knowledge with that of Medical Students and Pediatric Residents," *American Journal of Diseases of Children* 125 (February 1973):199–203; David L. Sackett, Walter O. Spitzer, Michael Gent and Robin S. Roberts, "The Burlington Randomized Trial of the Nurse Practitioner: Health Outcomes of Patients," *Annals of Internal Medicine* 80, no. 2 (February 1974):137–142; Walter O. Spitzer, David L. Sackett et al, "The Burlington Randomized Trial of the Nurse Practitioner," *New England Journal of Medicine* 290, no. 5 (January 31, 1974): 251–256.

Resource Document

"American Hospital Association Statement on the Role of the Physician's Assistant in the Hospital"*

PREAMBLE

Physician's assistants, functioning under the supervision of licensed physicians, possess potential for assisting in the delivery of high quality health care services in this country. Physician's assistants are currently working in health care institutions either as direct employees of the institution or as employees of physicians who maintain professional privileges in that institution. This fact, coupled with the increasing numbers of physician's assistants, suggests that the current American Hospital Association "Statement on the Physician's Assistant in the Hospital," dated November 18, 1970, should be replaced.

DEFINITION

Physician's assistants in the context of this document are members of the professional health care team, qualified by academic and clinical training, who perform certain assigned tasks ordinarily done by a physician and who work under the direction, supervision, and responsibility of a physician in accordance with policies established in medical staff bylaws of the health care institution. They exercise judgment within their areas of competence and participate directly in the medical care of patients under the supervision or direction of a member of the medical staff, performing functions to the extent delineated by the medical staff, such as compiling histories, giving physical examinations, and writing orders and recording progress notes on the physician's order and progress note forms.

---

*Approved by the American Hospital Association Council on Professional Services, March 7–8, 1974.

GENERAL INSTITUTIONAL POLICY

The medical staff and the administration should develop policies and procedures for recommendation to the governing body concerning the status, relationships, and functions of the physician's assistant in the institution, whether employed by a physician or by the institution. The policy should relate to both the general, overall utilization of physicians' assistants in the institution and to the utilization of each physician's assistant. Consultation with other appropriate relating disciplines at each institution should be sought when defining *general* policy. *General* policy should address at least the following issues:

1. Definition and classification of the scope of practice within the institution of different physician's assistants in accordance with their varying levels of competence and achievement.
2. Regulation or supervision of the physician's assistant by the sponsoring physician or a physician designee of the physician during the sponsor's absence. When a physician's assistant is employed by the institution there must be clear responsibility of a physician or his physician designee for the acts of the physician's assistant.
3. Identification of clinical procedures that require direct versus general supervision by the responsible physician, and appropriate methods of control by the institution.
4. Applications (or proposals) for the utilization of physician's assistants with the accompanying request for authorization to provide specified services should be processed by the credentials or other designated committee of the medical staff, which will make its recommendations to the chief executive officer. The qualifications of the sponsoring physician and his ability to provide supervision for the physician's assistant or assistants[1] for which he is responsible should be considered.
5. After employment by the physician or the health care institution, continuing utilization in the institution will be dependent upon ongoing evaluation by appropriate components of the medical staff and management.
6. When the physician's assistant is employed by the health care institution, the employment policies of the institution will prevail in addition to the foregoing professional review.

---

1. It should be noted that certain states limit the number of physician's assistants for which a physician may be responsible to two.

7. Suitable techniques for both verbal and visual identification of the physician's assistant to the patient, which make clear to the patient that he is not a physician, should be devised.
8. The mechanism for reduction or retraction of the functions and the patient care services the physician's assistant is permitted to perform and, in situations where the physician's assistant is an institutional employee, his dismissal from employment.
9. A mechanism for channeling physician's assistant grievances.
10. Responsibility for adequate liability insurance coverage for actions of the physician's assistant.
11. A system of continuing review and evaluation of the above issues.

POLICIES RELATING TO THE INDIVIDUAL

Policies for each individual physician's assistant should address at least the following issues:

1. Designation of the primarily responsible physician and a physician designee to function during his or her absence.
2. Assessment of the physician's assistant's credentials and continuing staff and institutional monitoring of each individual's performance.
3. The determination of the specific procedures and functions that each individual may be authorized to carry out in the institution pursuant to a professional review by the medical staff of the training, experience, demonstrated competence, and other pertinent qualifications of the prospective physician's assistant. The performance of these tasks must be subject to continuing review and evaluation by the medical staff. Considerations should include:
   a. the physician's assistant's eligibility for taking or successfully completing the National Board of Medical Examiner's Certifying Examination;
   b. the accreditation status of the physician's assistant training program from which the physician's assistant was graduated;[2]
   c. the specialty nature of the physician's assistant's academic and clinical training;
   d. state certification or licensure where required.

---

2. Listed by AMA publications and speciality societies.

LEGAL

There is a clear distinction between a physician's use of a physician's assistant in his private office and the use of the physician's assistant within the health care institution. In the one case only the physician, the patient, and the physician's assistant have an interest. When the physician's assistant performs functions within the institution as an employee either of the physician or of the institution, the institution is legally responsible. Therefore, in addition to the policy that the institution must develop, adopt, and implement with respect both to the general utilization of physician's assistants and the regulation of each particular physician's assistant, there must be awareness of the legal implications associated with the use of such individuals in the institution. This awareness must be a continuing concern of the institution because the institution is legally responsible for the selection, supervision, and working relationships of those persons who render care to patients whether or not those persons are employees.

The institution must, therefore, at all times exercise authority over the use of physician's assistants. Each physician's assistant must meet and continue to meet the institution's standards as well as those of the responsible physician. The activities of the physician's assistant must be monitored routinely and assessed periodically. By adopting and enforcing strict control procedures, the institution will meet its overall legal responsibility for the quality of care delivered to its patients.

At the present time, the statutes, cases, and regulations specifically relating to physician's assistants give little guidance to the institution that permits or plans to permit the use of these persons within its walls. Thus, the decision to permit physician's assistants to be used in the institution as employees either of a physician or of the institution must be made only after careful evaluation of their usefulness to the institution and only after serious evaluation of the legal risks and implications. If the institution decides to permit the use of physician's assistants, the functions that they will be permitted to perform must be strictly circumscribed, clearly spelled out, and effectively enforced. They must be strictly circumscribed so that the institution's legal risk is limited. They must be clearly delineated so that the physician sponsor or designee, employees, members of the medical staff, and the physician's assistant may know what the assistant is permitted to do. They must be effectively enforced so that problems can be avoided.

Legal counsel must play a major role in the development of institutional policy, rules, and regulations with respect to the use of physician's assistants in the institution. That policy must be based upon the current laws, regulations, and legal precedents of the state in which the institution is located. The institution, through its counsel, must consider at least the following issues:

1. Is there a state law[3] recognizing physician's assistants? What requirements does it impose concerning licensure, certification, training, and supervision of the physician's assistant?
2. Does the law specifically authorize or prohibit the hiring or utilization of physician's assistants?[4]
3. Do the state laws authorizing the practice of medicine, nursing, pharmacy, optometry, and other health professions bar any of the activities that a physician's assistant might be permitted to perform in the institution?
4. Does the institution's current public liability protection cover the use of physician's assistants?

---

3. Pertinent actions of the various regulatory agencies must be considered. The lack of specific legal authorization does not preclude the use of physician's assistants in the hospital.
4. The lack of specific legal authorization does not preclude the institution's hiring them.

"American Nurses' Association Definition of Nurse Practitioner, Nurse Clinician, and Clinical Nurse Specialist"*

The many terms to describe nurses who give care to patients have proliferated in the past several years. This proliferation can be related to the advancements of nursing theory and technology as well as to the desire for nurses to identify more specifically what they have become qualified to practice. Unfortunately, rather than clarifying nursing practice, all these terms and definitions have had a tendency to confuse levels of practice within the nursing profession as well as for other professions and consumers.

The Congress for Nursing Practice has been asked to clarify some of these definitions. This is no small task. It is a complicated task for several reasons. One, several state organizations or state councils on practice have already defined terminology for nurses. These definitions are not always compatible. Two, different parts of the country have different terminology. Three, those nurses practicing have definite opinions about how they wish their roles in practice to be defined. Four, health agencies, other professions, and educational institutions frequently have defined these terms in an effort to describe employment positions or set up curriculum. Five, there is a lack of uniformity in role requirements from agency to agency, and even within agencies.

The Congress for Nursing Practice presents the following definitions, which it believes constitute the first step toward an orderly process to insure uniformity of definitions for practitioners, employers, and consumers. The congress realizes that these definitions undoubtedly will have to be updated in the future to accommodate progress in the health care field.

---

*ANA Congress for Nursing Practice, May 8, 1974.

ROLES IN PRACTICE

Practitioners of professional nursing are registered nurses who provide direct care to clients utilizing the nursing process in arriving at decisions. They work in a collegial and collaborative relationship with other health professionals to determine health care needs and assume responsibility for nursing care. In the course of their practice they assess the effectiveness of actions taken, identify and carry out systematic investigations of clinical problems, and engage in periodic review of their own contributions to health care and those of their professional peers. In addition:

Nurse Practitioners have advanced skills in the assessment of the physical and psychosocial health-illness status of individuals, families, or groups in a variety of settings through health and development history-taking and physical examination. They are prepared for these special skills by formal continuing education which adheres to ANA approved guidelines, or in a baccalaureate nursing program.

Nurse Clinicians have well-developed competencies in utilizing a broad range of cues. These cues are used for prescribing and implementing both direct and indirect nursing care and for articulating nursing therapies with other planned therapies. Nurse clinicians demonstrate expertise in nursing practice and ensure ongoing development of expertise through clinical experience and continuing education. Generally minimal preparation for this role is the baccalaureate degree.

Clinical Nurse Specialists are primarily clinicians with a high degree of knowledge, skill, and competence in a specialized area of nursing. These are made directly available to the public through the provision of nursing care to clients and indirectly available through guidance and planning of care with other nursing personnel. Clinical nurse specialists hold a master's degree in nursing, preferably with an emphasis in clinical nursing.

Resource Document

"Nurses, in the Extended Role, are not Physician's Assistants"*

Nurses recently have been invited to participate in the Physician's Assistant Certification Program of the National Board of Medical Examiners. As a result of this invitation, ANA members have asked for clarification of the differences between the physician's assistant and the nurse practitioner.

In 1970 the American Medical Association Board of Trustees defined the physician's assistant: "The physician's assistant is a skilled person qualified by academic and practical training to provide patient services under the supervision and direction of a licensed physician *who is responsible for the performance of that assistant.*" In 1971 the ANA Board of Directors stated, "the term physician's assistant should not be applied to any of the nurse practitioners being prepared to function in an extension of the nursing role."

The basic length of preparation for a physician's assistant generally ranges between four months and four years. Currently, these programs are not evaluated, not standardized, and not accredited. Accreditation is a process by which an agency or organization evaluates and recognizes an institution or program of study as meeting certain predetermined criteria standards. Recently the AMA has begun the process of accrediting some of the physician assistants programs. On the other hand, a nurse has completed a basic nursing program which has been evaluated and approved by the board of nursing in the respective state, and, in addition, been accredited, in most instances, by the National League for Nursing. To become a practitioner, the nurse has acquired increased knowledge and clinical experience in a formal education program.

---

*ANA Statement released on July 9, 1973.

The term "nurse practitioner" refers to one who has completed the program of study leading to competence as a registered nurse in an expanded role whose responsibility encompasses:

1. obtaining a health history;
2. assessing health-illness status;
3. entering a person into the health care system;
4. sustaining and supporting persons who are impaired, infirm, or ill and during programs of diagnosis and therapy.

Selected Bibliography

FIRST EDITION—1972

Chapter One
Introduction

Andreoli, K. G. April 1972. A Look at the Physician's Assistant. *American Journal of Nursing* 72, no. 4: 710–13.

Carnegie Commission on Higher Education. 1970. *Higher Education and the Nation's Health: Policies for Medical and Dental Education.* New York: McGraw-Hill.

Dube, W. F.; Stritter, F. T.; Nelson, B. C. October 1971. Study of U.S. Medical School Applicants, 1970–71. *Journal of Medical Education* 46, no. 10:837–57.

Dublin, T. D. April 20, 1972. The Migration of Physicians to the United States. *New England Journal of Medicine* 286, no. 16:870–77.

Lewis, C.; Resnik, B.; Schmidt, G.; Waxman, D. March 20, 1969. Activities, Events and Outcomes in Ambulatory Patient Care. *New England Journal of Medicine* 280, no. 12:645–49.

McCormack, R.; Crawford, R. November–December, 1969. Attitudes of Professional Nurses Toward Primary Care. *Nursing Research* 18 no. 6:542–44.

Pascasio, A. March 1969. Continuing Education for Quality Health Care. *Physical Therapy* 49, no. 3:257–64.

Pondy, L. R. April 1970. Physician's Assistant Productivity: Ayden, North Carolina. Unpublished. Duke University, Durham, North Carolina.

Rogers, K. D.; Mally, M.; Marcus, F.; November 18, 1968. A General Medical Practice Using Nonphysician Personnel. *Journal of the American Medical Association* 206, no. 8:1753–57.

Rosinski, E.; Spencer, F. 1965. *The Assistant Medical Officer.* Chapel Hill, North Carolina: University of North Carolina Press.

Smith, R. A. 1969. Medex—A Demonstration Program in Primary Medical Care. *Northwest Medicine* 68:1023–30.

Stead, E. A. January 1967. The Duke Plan for Physician's Assistants. *Medical Times* 95, no. 1:40–48.

U.S. Civil Service Commission. March 1971. *Bridging the Medical Care Gap.* Announcement no. 428.

Veterans Administration. 1971. *Physician's Assistants—Guidelines for Utilization.* Circular no. 10–71–32.

Yankauer, A.; Connelly, J. P.; Feldman, J. J. July 1969. Task Performance and Task Delegation in Pediatric Office Practice. *American Journal of Public Health* 59, no. 7:1104–07.

Yankauer, A.; Connelly, J. P.; Feldman, J. J. January–February 1970. Physician Productivity in the Delivery of Ambulatory Care. *Medical Care* 8, no. 1:35–46.

Chapter Two
Some Fundamental Concerns

American Medical News. February 9, 1970. AMA Urges Major New Role for Nurses.

American Nurses' Association and the American Academy of Pediatrics (joint statement). January 1971. Guidelines on Short-Term Continuing Education Programs for Pediatric Nurse Associates.

Anderson, K. H.; Powers, L. January 1970. The Pediatric Assistant. *North Carolina Medical Journal* 31, no. 1:1–8.

Andreoli, K. G.; Stead, E. A. July 1967. Training Physician's Assistants at Duke. *American Journal of Nursing* 67, no. 7:1442–43.

Andrews, P.; Yankauer, A.; Connelly, J. May 1970. Changing the Patterns of Ambulatory Pediatric Caretaking—An Action-Oriented Training Program for Nurses. *American Journal of Public Health* 60:870–79.

Cain, R.; Kohn, J. November 1971. Pharmacist as a Member of the Health Team. *American Journal of Public Health* 61, no. 11:2223–28.

Carlson, C. L., Athelstan, G. T. December 7, 1970. The Physician's Assistant: Versions and Diversions of a Promising Concept. *Journal of the American Medical Association* 214, no. 10:1855–61.

Charney, E.; Kitzman, H. In Collaboration with Berkow, E.; Cafarelli, C.; Davis, L.; Disney, R.; Friedlander, C.; Green, J.; Hare, N.; MacWhinney, J.; Miller, R. December 9, 1971. The Child-Health Nurse (Pediatric Nurse Practitioner) in Private Practice. *The New England Journal of Medicine* 285, no. 24:1353–58.

Coye, R.; Hansen, M. July 28, 1969. The Doctor's Assistant: A Survey of Physicians' Expectations. *Journal of the American Medical Association* 209, no.4:529–33.

Crook, W. November 1969. A Practicing Pediatrician Looks at Associates, Assistants, and Aides. *Pediatric Clinics of North America* 16, no. 4:929–38.

Darley, E.; Somers, A. R. June 8, 1967. Medicine, Money and Manpower—The Challenge to Professional Education (II. Opportunity for New Excellence). *New England Journal of Medicine* 276, no. 23:1291–96.

Duncan, B.; Smith, A.; Silver, H. March 1970. Comparison of the Physical Assessment of Children by Pediatric Nurse Practitioners and Pediatricians. Mimeographed. University of Colorado.

Egeberg. R. O. October 1970. Allied Health Workers—Now and Tomorrow. *Manpower* 2, no. 10:3–7.

Eisenberg, H. May 15, 1967. How an R.N. Midwife Can Help. *Medical Economics* 44, no. 2:78–83.

Estes, E. H. June 29, 1970. The Training of Physician's Assistants: A New Challenge for Medical Education. *Modern Medicine* 38:90–93.

Estes, E. H.; Howard, D. R. March 1970. Potential for Newer Classes of Personnel: Experiences of the Duke Physician's Assistant Program. *Journal of Medical Education* 45, no. 3:149–55.

Fein, R. 1967. *The Doctor Shortage: An Economic Diagnosis.* Washington, D.C.: Brookings Institution.

Fendall, N. May–June 1968. The Auxiliary In Medicine. *Israel Journal of Medical Science* 4, no. 3:614–28.

Ginzberg, E. July 14, 1966. Physician Shortage Reconsidered. *New England Journal of Medicine* 275, no. 2:85–87.

Greenberg, S.; Galton, R. February 1972. Nurses are Key in HIP Experiment to Cut Health Care Costs. *American Journal of Nursing* 72, no. 2:272–76.

Health Manpower Source Book. 1969. *Manpower Supply and Educational Statistics for Selected Health Occupations.* Washington, D.C.: U.S. Government Printing Office.

Ingles, T. May 1968. A New Health Worker. *American Journal of Nursing* 68 no. 5:1059–61.

Josiah Macy Jr. Foundation. 1970. *The Training and Utilization of Pediatric Assistants.* Report of Conference, Williamsburg, Virginia, December 10–12, 1969. New York: Macy Foundation.

Journal of the American Medical Association. March 10, 1969. New Mexico Hamlet Avoids Medical Isolation. 207, no. 10:1808–09.

Kadish, J.; Long, J. May 11, 1970. The Training of Physician Assistants: Status and Issues. *Journal of the American Medical Association* 212, no. 6:1047–51.

Kaku, K.; Gilbert, F. I.; Sachs, R. R. December 1970. Comparison of Health Appraisals by Nurses and Physicians. *Public Health Reports* 85, no. 12:1042–46.

Knowles, J. H. February 1969. The Quantity and Quality of Medical Manpower: A Review of Medicine's Current Efforts. *Journal of Medical Education* 44 no. 2:81–118.

Lewis, C.; Resnik, B. December 7, 1967. Nurse Clinics and Progressive Ambulatory Patient Care. *New England Journal of Medicine* 277, no. 23:236–41.

Lewis, E. 1970. *The Clinical Nurse Specialist.* New York: The American Journal of Nursing Company.

Medical World News. November 19, 1971. Setback for Medex Programs. 12, no. 43:83–84.

Mereness, D. May 1970. Recent Trends in Expanding Roles of the Nurse. *Nursing Outlook* 18, no. 5:30–33.

Montgomery, T. October 1, 1969. A Case for Nurse-Midwives. *American Journal of Obstetrics and Gynecology* 105:309–13.

Myers, H. September 1969. The Physician's Assistant. *West Virginia Medical Journal* 65, no. 9:303–04.

Nursing Outlook. January 1972. Preparing Nurses for Family Health Care. 20, no. 1:53–59.

Obrig. A. May 1971. A Nurse-Midwife in Practice. *American Journal of Medicine* 71 no. 5:953–57.

Oseasohn, R.; Mortimer, E. A.; Geil, C. C.; Eberle, B. J.; Pressman, A. E.; Quenk, N. L. November 29, 1971. Rural Medical Care: Physician's Assistant Linked to an Urban Medical Center. *Journal of the American Medical Association* 218, no. 9:1417–19.

Patterson, P.; Skinner, A. February 1971. Physician Response to Delegation of Well Child Care. *Northwest Medicine* 70, no. 2:92–96.

Riddick, F. A.; Bryan J. B.; Gershenson, M. I.; Costello, A. C. May 1971. Use of Allied Health Professionals in Internists' Offices. *Archives of Internal Medicine* 127, no. 5:924–31.

Schiff, D. W.; Fraser, C. H., Walters, H. L. July 1969. The Pediatric Nurse Practitioner in the Office of Pediatricians in Private Practice. *Pediatrics* 44, no. 1:62–68.

Schulman, J.; Wood, C. March 13, 1972. Experience of a Nurse Practitioner in a General Medicine Clinic. *Journal of the American Medical Association* 219, no. 11:1453–61.

Sidel, V. W. April 25, 1968. Feldshers and 'Feldsherism.' *New England Journal of Medicine* 278, no. 17:934–39.

Sidel, V. W. May 2, 1968. Feldshers and 'Feldsherism' (Concluded). *New England Journal of Medicine* 278, no. 18:987–92.

Silver, H. K. May 24, 1971. The School Nurse Practitioner Program. *Journal of the American Medical Association* 216, no. 8:1332–34.

Silver, H. K. September 6, 1971. The Syniatrist. *Journal of the American Medical Association* 217, no. 10:1368–70.

Silver, H. K.; Ford, L. C.; Day, L. R. April 22, 1968. The Pediatric Nurse-Practitioner Program: Expanding the Role of the Nurse to Provide Increased Health Care for Children. *Journal of the American Medical Association* 204:298–302.

Silver, H. K.; Ford, L. C.; Stearly, S. C. May 1967. A Program to Increase Health Care for Children: The Pediatric Nurse Practitioner Program. *Pediatrics* 39, no. 5:756–60.

Silver, H. K.; Hecker, J. A. March 1970. The Pediatric Nurse Practitioner and the Child Health Associate: New Types of Health Professionals. *Journal of Medical Education* 45 no. 3:171–76.

Silver H. K.; McAtee, P. A. January 1972. Health Care Practice: An Expanded Profession of Nursing for Men and Women. *American Journal of Nursing* 72 no. 1:78–80.

Skinner, A. May 1968. Parental Acceptance of Delegated Pediatric Services. *Pediatrics* 41, no. 5:1003–04.

Smith R. A. March 16, 1970. MEDEX. *Journal of the American Medical Association* 211, no. 16:1843–45.

Smith, R. A.; Bassett, G. R.; Markarian, C. A.; Vath, R. E.; Freeman, W. L.; Dunn, G. F. September 6, 1971. A Strategy for Health Manpower: Reflections on an Experience Called MEDEX. *Journal of the American Medical Association* 217, no. 10:1362–67.

Stead, E. A. December 5, 1966. Conserving Costly Talents—Providing Physician's New Assistants. *Journal of the American Medical Association* 198, no. 10:1108–09.

Stead, E. A. February 1967. At Duke: A New Approach to the Doctor Shortage. *Resident Physician* 13:84–96.

Stead, E. A. October 1967. Current Concepts: Training and Use of Paramedical Personnel. *New England Journal of Medicine* 277 no. 15:800–01.

U.S. Department of Health, Education and Welfare. May 1971. *Towards a Comprehensive Health Policy for the 1970s: A White Paper.* Washington: U.S. Government Printing Office.

Walker, A. E. January 1972. PRIMEX—The Family Nurse Practitioner Program. *Nursing Outlook* 20, no. 1:28–31.

Weed, L. L. March 14, 1968. Medical Records that Guide and Teach. *New England Journal of Medicine* 278, no. 11:593–600.

Wisconsin Medical Journal. January 1969. Physician's Guidelines for Delegation of Duties and Functions to Nurses. 68:42–43.

Wise, H. January 1971. Social Problems Facing Medicine—Invert and Proceed. *Archives of Internal Medicine* 127:76–79.

Yankauer, A.; Connelly, J. P.; Feldman, J. November 1968. A Survey of Allied Health Worker Utilization in Pediatric Practice in Massachusetts and the U.S. *Pediatrics* 42, no. 5:733–42.

Yankauer, A.; Connelly, J. P.; Feldman, J. J. January–February 1970. Physician Productivity in the Delivery of Ambulatory Care. *Medical Care* VIII, no. 1:35–46.

Yankauer, A.; Connelly, J. P.; Feldman, J. J. March 1970 (supplement). Pediatric Practices in the United States with Special Attention to Utilization of Allied Health Worker Services. *Pediatrics*,45 sup:521–54.

Chapter Three
Lessons from Nursing

Aisen, M. W. December 1970. Up the Vocational Stairs. *American Journal of Nursing* 70, no. 12:2614–17.

Alden, V. September 1, 1971. How Much Is College Education Worth? *Wall Street Journal.*

American Journal of Nursing. April 1970. AMA Unveils Surprise Plan to Convert R.N. into Medic. 70, no. 4:691.

American Journal of Nursing. May 1970. Nurse Groups Ask R.N.–M.D. Dialogue, Some Get It. 70, no. 5:953–54.

American Journal of Nursing. May 1971. Dearth of Nursing Research Concerns Researchers at ANA Sponsored Session. 71, no. 5:878.

American Nurses Association Position Paper. 1965. Educational Preparation for Nurse Practitioners and Assistants to Nurses.

Bailey, D. H. 1969. Nursing in Transition. International Nursing Review 18, no. 1:59–65.

Bates, B. July 16, 1970. Doctor and Nurse: Changing Roles and Relations. New England Journal of Medicine 283:129.

Beal, J. February 1971. This I Believe . . . About the National League for Nursing. Nursing Outlook 19, no. 2:99–102.

Bennett, L. R. January 1970. This I Believe . . . That Nurses May Become Extinct. Nursing Outlook. 18:28–32.

Bennis, W.; Berkowitz, N.; Malone, M.; Klein, M. 1961. The Role of the Nurse in the Out-Patient Department. New York: American Nurses Foundation.

Bergman, A. May 1971. Physician's Assistants Belong in the Nursing Profession. American Journal of Nursing 71, no. 5:975–77.

Blum, H. March 15–17, 1971. Barriers to Manpower Mobility and Utilization: Paper prepared for National Health Council Meeting.

Christy, T.; Poulin, M.; Hover, J. August 1971. An Appraisal of An Abstract for Action. American Journal of Nursing 71, no. 8:1574–81.

Courtney, M. May 1971. Nursing Education, The Diploma Programs. RN 34, no. 5:37–39, 58–64.

DeChow, G. May 1971. Nursing Education, The Associate Degree Programs. RN 34, no. 5:41–43, 66–75.

deTornyay, R. May 1971. Expanding the Nurse's Role Does Not Make Her a Physician's Assistant. American Journal of Nursing 71, no. 5:974–76.

Dilworth, A. September 1970. Joint Preparation for Clinical Nurse Specialists. Nursing Outlook 18, no. 9:22–25.

DuMouchell, N. November 1970. Are We Really Meeting our Patients' Needs? The Canadian Nurse 66, no. 11:39–43.

Estes, E. H. June 1969. Task Oriented vs. Degree Oriented Training Concept of Optimizing the Use of the Most Highly Skilled with Specific Personnel. Military Medicine 134:386–89.

Frank, L. 1969. Fragmentation in the Helping Professions. In Bennis, W.; Benne, K.; Chin, R. The Planning of Change, pp. 43–48. New York: Holt, Rinehart and Winston.

Ginzberg, E. 1969. Men, Money and Medicine. New York: Columbia University Press.

Golub, J. August 16, 1971. A Nurse-Internship Program. Hospitals, JAHA 45:73–78.

Hale, T. November 10, 1966. Problems of Supply and Demand in the Education of Nurses. The New England Journal of Medicine 275, no. 19: 1044–48.

Hale, T. April 18, 1968. Cliches of Nursing Education. New England Journal of Medicine 278, no. 16:879–86.

Heckinger, R. August 1971. It's Time to Amalgamate Our Educational System. *RN* 34, no. 8:42–45.

Herzberg, F.; Mausner, B.; Snyderman, B. 1959. *The Motivation to Work.* New York: John Wiley and Sons.

HEW Bureau of Health Manpower, Division of Nursing. December 1967. *Nurse Training Act of 1964 Program Review Report,* Public Health Service pub. no. PHS–1740.

HEW Public Health Service, Report of the Surgeon General's Consultant Group on Nursing. 1963. *Toward Quality in Nursing,* PHS–992.

Hospitals, JAHA. January 1, 1972. Hospital Schools of Nursing: 'Alive and Kicking.' 46, no. 1:56–63.

Hudson, B. September 1971. The Medical Student As A Nurse's Assistant. *Journal of Medical Education* 46:791–92.

Ingles, T. June 1971. Mobility in Nursing. *Rhode Island Medical Journal* 54:313–15.

Kibrick, A. April 4, 1968. Why Collegiate Programs for Nurses? *New England Journal of Medicine* 278, no. 14:765–72.

Kramer, M.; Baker, C. May–June 1971. The Exodus: Can We Prevent It? *Journal of Nursing Administration* 1, no. 3:15–29.

Krueger, J. C. October 1971. The Education and Utilization of Nurses: A Paradox. *Nursing Outlook* 19, no. 10:676–79.

Lambertsen, E. C. December 1, 1971. Nursing: Not Quite M.D., More Than P.A. *Hospitals, JAHA* 45, no. 23:70–76.

Lambertsen, E. C. January 1972. Perspective on the Physician's Assistant. *Nursing Outlook* 20, no. 1:32–36.

Levine, E. February 1969. Nurse Manpower, Yesterday, Today, and Tomorrow. *American Journal of Nursing* 69, no. 2:290–96.

Lewis, E., ed. 1971. *Changing Patterns of Nursing Practice.* New York: American Journal of Nursing Company.

Lockerby, F. K. December 1971. Nurses' Role Expanded. *Hospitals, JAHA* 45, no. 24:92–98.

MacGregor, F. December 12, 1966. Nursing in Transition. *Journal of the American Medical Association* 198, no. 11:174–75.

McIntyre, H. M. January 1971. The Nurse—Technical Assistant or Professional Associate? *Chest* 59, no. 1:3–4.

Maslow, A. 1970. *Motivation and Personality.* 2nd ed. New York: Harper and Row.

Mauksch, I. February 1971. This I Believe . . . About the National League for Nursing. *Nursing Outlook* 19, no. 2:98–101.

Medical World News. February 13, 1970. Nurses Play MD? It's News to Them, p. 15.

Medical World News. January 14, 1972. A Nurse By Any Other Name, pp. 73–75.

Mereness, D. May 1971. Nursing Education, The Baccalaureate and Higher Degree Programs. *RN* 34, no. 5:44–47, 80–82.

National Commission for the Study of Nursing and Nursing Education. 1970. *An Abstract for Action.* New York: McGraw–Hill.

National Commission for the Study of Nursing and Nursing Education. 1970.
Nurse Clinician and Physician's Assistant: The Relationship Between
Two Emerging Practitioner Concepts. Brochure.
Nursing Research. May–June, 1971. Research in Nursing—A Critical Need. 20,
no. 3.
Paynich, M. L. April 1971. Why Do Basic Nursing Students Work in Nursing?
Nursing Outlook 19, no. 4:242–45.
Pearlmutter, D. R.; Warner, G. M. November 15, 1970. Attitudes of Physicians
to Nurses. *New York State Journal of Medicine* 70, no. 22:2840–46.
Robinson, A. M. March 1972. The R.N.: Without Her, No ICUs. *RN* 35:46–52.
Rogers, M. E. January 1972. Nursing: To Be or Not To Be? *Nursing Outlook* 20,
no. 1:42–46.
Shaw, B. June 1971. The Nurse-PA: One Experiment That's Working! *RN* 34,
no. 6:45–47.
Smith, E. February 1, 1972. RN Graduates: Where Do They Go? *Hospitals,
JAHA* 46:136–42.

Chapter Four
Where the Law Intervenes
American Hospital Association, Special Committee on Licensure of Health
Personnel. Approved November 18, 1970. Statement on Licensure
of Health Personnel. Mimeographed.
American Medical Association, Committee on Nursing. September 14, 1970.
Medicine and Nursing in the 1970s—A Position Statement. *Journal
of the American Medical Association* 213, no. 11:1881–83.
American Medical Association, Council on Health Manpower. Adopted December 1970. Licensure of Health Occupations. Mimeographed.
Anderson, B. February 7, 1969. Licensure of Paramedical Personnel. Paper
presented at the 65th Annual Meeting of the Federation of State
Medical Boards of the United States.
Ballenger, M. May 17, 1971. Current Efforts to Implement the Physician's
Assistant Concept. *Modern Medicine* 39, no. 10:65–89.
Ballenger, M.; Estes, E. H. 1969. *Model Legislation Project for Physician's Assistants* Durham, N.C.: Duke University, Department of Community
Health Sciences.
Carlson, R. J. Autumn 1970. Health Manpower Licensing and Emerging Institutional Responsibility for the Quality of Care. *Law & Contemporary
Problems* 35, no. 4:849–78.
Connecticut Medicine. August 1971. Forewarned is Forearmed: Governor Signs
Physician's Assistant Bill. 35, no. 2:78–80.
Curran, W. J. May 7, 1970. New Paramedical Personnel—To License or Not to
License? *New England Journal of Medicine* 282, no. 19:1085–86.
Curran, W. J. December 3, 1970. The California 'Physicians' Assistants' Law.
New England Journal of Medicine 283, no. 23:1274–75.
Curran, W. J. February 3, 1972. Legal Responsibility for Actions of Physicians'
Assistants. *New England Journal of Medicine* 286, no. 5:254.

Derbyshire, R. C. *1969. Medical Licensure and Discipline in the United States.* Baltimore: Johns Hopkins Press.

Driscoll, V. January 1972. Liberating Nursing Practice. *Nursing Outlook* 20, no. 1:24–28.

Forgotson, E.; Bradley, C.; Ballenger, M. December 1970. Health Services for the Poor—The Manpower Problem: Innovations and the Law. *Wisconsin Law Review* 1970, no. 3:756–89.

Forgotson, E. H.; Forgotson, J. January–February 1970. Innovations and Experiments in Uses of Health Manpower. *Medical Care* 8, no. 1:3–14.

Hammond, K. R.; Kelly, K. J.; Schneider, R. J.; Vancini. Spring 1966. Clinical Inference in Nursing. *Nursing Research* 15:134–38.

Havighurst, C. C. November 13, 1970. "Licensure and its Alternatives." The Third Annual Duke Conference on Physician's Assistants, pp. 121–31. Available from the Department of Community Health Sciences, Duke University, Durham, N.C.

Hershey, N. 1955. *Toward Better Definition of Nursing.* Pittsburgh, Pa.: University of Pittsburgh Health Law Center, Graduate School of Public Health.

Hershey, N. March 1969. An Alternative to Mandatory Licensure of Health Professionals. *Hospital Progress* 50:71–73.

Hershey, N. January 1972. Standards of Performance in Expanded Practice. *American Journal of Nursing* 72, no. 1:86–87.

Kaplan, W. A. 1972. The Law's View of Professional Power: Courts and the Health Professional Associations. *SASHEP Staff Working Papers*, vol. 2.

Kaplan, W. A.; Hunter J. P. 1966. The Legal Status of the Educational Accrediting Agency: Problems in Judicial Supervision and Governmental Regulation. *Cornell Law Quarterly* 52:104–31.

Kinlein, M. L. January 1972. Independent Nurse Practitioner. *Nursing Outlook* 20, no. 1:22–24.

Leff, A. Summer 1967. Medical Devices and Paramedical Personnel: A Preliminary Context for Emerging Problems. *Washington University Law Quarterly*, 1967, no. 3:332–413.

Lesnik, M. J.; Anderson, B. E. *1955. Nursing Practice and the Law.* Philadelphia: J. B. Lippincott.

Murray, B. L. January 1972. A Case for Independent Group Nursing Practice. *Nursing Outlook* 20, no. 1:60–63.

Newman, F. 1971. *Report on Higher Education* (to the Secretary of Health, Education and Welfare). Washington, D.C.: U.S. Government Printing Office.

Note. 1968. Acts of Diagnosis by Nurses and the Colorado Professional Nursing Act. *Denver Law Journal* 45:467–89.

Nursing Outlook. January 1972. Extending the Scope of Nursing Practice. 20, no. 1:46–52.

Patterson, P.K.; Bergman, A. B.; Wedgwood, R. J. July, 1969. Parent Reaction to the Concept of Pediatric Assistants. *Pediatrics.* 44 no. 1:69–75.

Pennell, M. Y.; Proffitt, J. R.; Hatch, T. 1971. The Role of Professional Associations in the Regulation of Health Manpower through Accreditation and Certification. *1971 National Health Forum*, "Health Manpower: Adapting in the Seventies," pp. 53–78.

Pennell, M. Y.; Hoover, D. B. February 1972. Policies for the Development of Credentialing Mechanisms for Health Personnel. *Operation MEDIHC Newsletter 2*, no. 3. Published by the National Health Council, New York.

Report of the National Advisory Commission on Health Manpower. Vols. 1 and 2. Washington, D.C., 1967(I), 1968(II).

Roemer, R. January–February 1971. Licensing and Regulation of Medical and Medical-Related Practitioners in Health Service Teams. *Medical Care 9*, no. 1:42–54.

Roemer, R. March 15, 1971. Legal Regulation of Health Manpower in the 1970s: Needs, Objectives, Options, Constraints, and their Trade-Offs. *1971 National Health Forum.*

Sadler, A. M. Jr.; Sadler, B. L. July 1970. Licensure and Certification of Health Personnel. A Report to the Assistant Secretary for Health and Scientific Affairs, HEW. Unpublished.

Sadler, A. M. Jr.; Sadler, B. L. November 1971. Recent Developments in the Law Relating to the Physician's Assistant. *Vanderbilt Law Review 24*, no. 6:1193–1212.

Selden, W. January 1970. Licensing Boards are Archaic. *American Journal of Nursing 70*, no. 1:124–26.

Silver, H. April 22, 1968. The Pediatric Nurse Practitioner Program. *Journal of the American Medical Association 204*, no. 4:298–302.

Silver, H. February 11, 1971. New Allied Health Professionals: Implications of the Colorado Child Health Associate Law. *New England Journal of Medicine 284*, no. 6:304–07.

Stevens, R. 1971. *American Medicine and the Public Interest.* New Haven: Yale University Press.

Stead, E. A. November 12, 1970. "Dependence vs. Independence and its Relationship to the Professional Physician's Assistant." Third Annual Duke Conference on Physician's Assistants. Available from the Department of Community Health Sciences, Duke University, Durham, N.C.

Study for the Accreditation of Selected Health Education Programs. May 1972. *Commission Report.* Washington, D.C.: National Commission on Accreditation.

Study of Accreditation of Selected Health Educational Programs. October 1971. *Part One: Working Papers.* Washington, D.C.: National Commission on Accrediting.

Study of Accreditation of Selected Health Educational Programs. February 1972. *Part Two: Staff Working Papers.* Washington, D.C.: National Commission on Accrediting.

U.S. Department of Health, Education and Welfare, Secretary's Committee Report. 1972. *Extending the Scope of Nursing Practice.* HEW pub.

no. 0-720-301. Washington, D.C.: U.S. Government Printing Office.
U.S. Department of Health, Education and Welfare (to the Congress of the United States). July 28, 1971. *Report on Licensure and Related Health Personnel Credentialing.* HEW pub. no. (ASM) 72-11.

Wald, F.; Leonard, R. 1964. Toward Development of Nursing Practice Theory. *Nursing Research* 13:309-13.

Young, L. S. January 1972. Physician's Assistants and the Law. *Nursing Outlook* 20 no. 1:36-41.

Chapter Five
Organizational Alternatives

Argyris, C. 1964. *Integrating the Individual and the Organization.* New York: John Wiley and Sons.

Beloff, J. S.; Korper, M. January 17, 1972. The Health Team Model and Medical Care Utilization. *Journal of the American Medical Association* 219, no. 3:359-66.

Bennis, W.; Benne, K.; Chin, R. 1961. *The Planning of Change.* New York: Holt, Rinehart and Winston.

Breytspraak, L.; Pondy, L. March 1969. Sociological Evaluation of the Physician's Assistants Role Relations. *Group Practice* 18, no. 3:32-41.

Duncan, B.; Kempe, C. November 1968. Joint Education of Medical Students and Allied Health Personnel. *Amer. J. Dis. Child.* 116:499-504.

Ledney, D. August 1971. Psychiatric Nursing: Breakthrough to Independence? *RN* 34, no. 8:29-35.

Likert, R. 1961. *New Patterns of Management.* New York: McGraw-Hill.

McGregor, D. 1960. *The Human Side of Enterprise.* New York: McGraw-Hill.

McGregor, D. 1966. *Leadership and Motivation.* Cambridge, Mass.: The MIT Press.

Novack, A. H.; Abramovitz, M. 1973. Primary Care Health Teams: An Annotated Bibliography. Prepared for the Maternal and Child Health Services, HEW, *HSMHA.*

Pellegrino, E. F. May 22, 1970. *The Changing Matrix of Clinical Decision-Making.* Ann Arbor, Mich.: University of Michigan Institute for Social Research Survey Research Center.

Pellegrino, E. F. 1972. Closing the 'Profession Gap'—Some Notes on Unity of Purpose in the Health Professions. In E. J. McTernan and R. O. Hawkins, eds., *Educating Personnel for the Allied Health Professions and Services: Administrative Considerations.* St. Louis: C. V. Mosby.

Schein, E. 1965. *Organizational Psychology.* Englewood Cliffs, N.J.: Prentice-Hall.

Schein, E.; Bennis, W. 1965. *Personal and Organizational Change Through Group Methods.* New York: John Wiley and Sons.

Wise, H. B. July 1968. Montefiore Hospital Neighborhood Medical Care Demonstration: A Case Study. *Milbank Memorial Fund Quarterly* 46: 297-307.

SECOND EDITION—1975

Alpert, J.; Charney, E. Autumn 1973. The Education of Physicians for Primary Care. U.S. DHEW Pub. No. (HRA) 74–3113.

American Academy of Physicians' Assistants and The Association of Physician Assistant Programs. 1974. *Proceedings of The Second National Conference on New Health Practitioners*, March 27–30, 1974, New Orleans, Louisiana. Baltimore: Williams and Wilkins.

Andreopoulos, S., ed. 1974. *Primary Care: Where Medicine Fails.* New York: John Wiley and Sons.

Andrus, L.; Geyman, J. 1973. Managing the Health Care Team. In Conn, Rakel, Johnson eds. *Family Practice*, ch. 10. Philadelphia: W. B. Saunders. See also, Fall 1973. *The P. A. Journal—A Journal for New Health Practitioners* 3, no. 4:5–22.

Appel, G. 1975. *Physician Extenders: An Evaluation of Policy-Related Research.* Minneapolis. InterStudy's Library.

Association of American Medical Colleges. 1974. *Proceedings of The Institute on Primary Care.* October 6–8, 1974. Washington, D.C.: Association of American Medical Colleges.

Association of Physician Assistant Programs. 1974. *National Physician Assistant Program. Profile 1975–76.* 1st ed. Washington, D.C.: Association of Physician Assistant Programs.

Baker, A. January 31, 1974. Primary Care by the Nurse. *New England Journal of Medicine* 290, no. 5:282–283.

Baker, C. March 1974. What's Different About Family Medicine? *Journal of Medical Education* 49, no. 3:231.

Bates, B. 1974. *A Guide to Physical Examination.* Philadelphia: J. B. Lippincott.

Beeson, P. January 1974. Some Good Features of the British National Health Service. *Journal of Medical Education* 49, no. 1:43–49.

Belknap, M.; Blau, R. A.; Grossman, R. N. 1975. *Case Studies and Methods in Humanistic Medical Care.* San Francisco: Institute for the Study of Humanistic Medicine.

Bjorn, J. June 1971. Physician's Assistant—Second Level Entrepreneur? *Journal of the Maine Medical Association* 62, no. 6:133–135, 144. See also, Fall 1973. *The P.A. Journal—A Journal for New Health Practitioners* 3, no. 4:28–31.

Bliss, A. Fall 1973. Interdependence: Changing Practice Styles for Improved Health Care. *The P.A. Journal—A Journal for New Health Practitioners* 3, no. 4:3–4.

Browning, M.; Lewis, E. eds. 1973. *The Expanded Role of the Nurse.* New York: The American Journal of Nursing Company.

Bullough, B.; St. Geme, J.; Neumann, C. October 1973. Pediatric Nurse Practitioners—Issues in Training. *Health Services Reports* 88, no. 8: 767–771.

Carlson, R. J. 1975. *The End of Medicine.* New York: John Wiley and Sons, Inc.

Center for Community Health Systems. 1975. *Community Hospitals and the Challenge of Primary Care.* New York: Columbia University.

Chappell, J.; Drogos, P. June 1972. Evaluation of Infant Health Care by a Nurse Practitioner. *Pediatrics* 49, no. 6:871–877.

Charney, E.; Kitzman, H. December 9, 1971. The Child-Health Nurse (Pediatric Nurse Practitioner) in Private Practice: A Controlled Trial. *New England Journal of Medicine* 285, no. 24:1353–1358.

Cohen, E. D. October 1974. *An Evaluation of Policy Related Research on New and Expanded Roles of Health Workers: Executive Summary.* New Haven: Yale University School of Medicine, Office of Regional Activities and Continuing Education.

Cohen, E. D. et al. October 1974. *An Evaluation of Policy Related Research on New and Expanded Roles of Health Workers.* New Haven: Yale University School of Medicine, Office of Regional Activities and Continuing Education.

Cohen, E. D. et al. October 1974. *An Evaluation of Policy Related Research on New and Expanded Roles of Health Workers: Annotated Bibliography.* New Haven: Yale University School of Medicine, Office of Regional Activities and Continuing Education.

Cohen, H. Winter 1973. Professional Licensure, Organizational Behavior and the Public Interest. *Milbank Memorial Fund Quarterly* 51, no. 1:73–88.

Conrad, M.; Fernald, L. Fall 1974. Nurses in Participatory Medicine: A Hidden Curriculum of Acquiescence? *The P.A. Journal—A Journal for New Health Practitioners* 4, no. 3:46–53.

Crichton, M. 1970. *Five Patients.* New York: Bantam.

Crovitz, E.; Huse, M.; Lewis, D. January 1973. Field Ratings of Physician's Assistants (Associates). *Physician's Associate* 3, no. 1:19–21.

Crovitz, E.; Huse, M.; Lewis, D. June 1973. Selection of Physician's Assistants. *Journal of Medical Education* 48:551–555.

deCastro, F. J.; Rolfe, U. T. February 1974. An Evaluation of New Primary Pediatric Paraprofessionals. *Journal of Medical Education* 49, no. 2:192–193. See also, Fall 1974. *The P.A. Journal—A Journal for New Health Practitioners* 4, no. 3:44–45.

Ebert, R. H. September 1973. The Medical School. *Scientific American* 229, no. 3:139–148.

Eichhorn, S. 1974. *Becoming: the actualization of individual differences in five student health teams.* Bronx, N.Y.: Institute for Health Team Development.

Fendall, N. 1972. *Auxiliaries in Health Care—Programs in Developing Countries.* Baltimore, Md.: The Johns Hopkins Press.

Fine, L. L.; Silver, H. K. August 1973. Comparative Diagnostic Abilities of Child Health Associate Interns and Practicing Pediatricians. *The Journal of Pediatrics* 83, no. 2:332–335.

Fisher, D. W. 1975. Physician Assistant—A Profile of the Profession. Presented at the 3rd Annual Conference on New Health Practitioners, St. Louis, April 7, 1975.

Ford, A. March 1975. *Physician Assistant—A National and Local Analysis.* New York: Praeger Publishers, Inc.

Frontier Nursing Service. 1975. *Medical Directives.* 7th Ed. Wendover, Ky.: Frontier Nursing Service.

Fuchs, V. R. 1974. *Who Shall Live—Health, Economics and Social Choice.* New York: Basic Books.

Golden, A.; Carlson, D.; and Harris, B. August 1973. Non-Physician Family Health Teams for Health Maintenance Organizations. *American Journal of Public Health* 63, no. 8:732–736.

Golladay, F.; Miller, M.; Smith, K. November–December 1973. Allied Health Manpower Strategies: Estimates of the Potential Gains from Efficient Task Delegation. *Medical Care* 11, no. 6:457–469.

Grimm, R.; Shimoni, K.; Harlan, W.; and Estes, E. March 6, 1975. Evaluation of Patient Care Protocol Use for Various Providers. *New England Journal of Medicine* 292, no. 10:507–511.

Halberstam, M. J. May 27, 1971. Liberal Thought, Radical Theory and Medical Practice. *New England Journal of Medicine* 284, no. 21:1180–1185.

Hawthorne, M.; Perry, W. 1974. *Community Colleges and Primary Health Care: Study of Allied Health Education (SAHE) Report.* Washington, D.C.: American Association of Community and Junior Colleges.

Heikkinen, C. November 1973. Open-Closed Mindedness and the Physician's Assistant: An Exploratory Study. *Journal of Medical Education* 48, no. 11:1013–1018.

Henry, R. A. October 1972. Use of Physician's Assistants in Gilchrist County, Florida. *Health Services Reports* 87, no. 8:687–692.

Hilmar, N.; McAtee, P. September 1973. The School Nurse Practitioner and Her Practice: A Study of Traditional and Expanded Health Care Responsibilities for Nurses in Elementary School. *Journal of School Health* 43, no. 7:431–441.

Illich, I. 1974. *Medical Nemesis.* London: Calder and Boyars.

Jewett, R. 1974. Response to a Paper by Dr. Charles E. Lewis on "Training the New Health Practitioner." *Proceedings of The Institute on Primary Care.* October 6–8, 1974. Washington, D.C.: Association of American Medical Colleges.

Kacen, A. July 1972. A Social Viewpoint of the Physician's Assistant Movement, Part I. *Physician's Associate* 2, no. 3:83–88.

Kacen, A. January 1973. The Physician Assistant: An Added Impetus to Excellence in Nursing. *Physician's Associate* 3, no. 1:9–13.

Kacen, A. April 1973. The Physician's Assistant Movement: Potential Impetus for a Competency-Based Medical School Curriculum. *The P.A. Journal—A Journal for New Health Practitioners* 3, no. 2:6–10.

Kindig, D. 1974. Primary Health Care Teams: Issues for Team Delivery and Interdisciplinary Education. *Proceedings of The Institute on Primary Care.* October 6–8, 1974. Washington, D.C.: Association of American Medical Colleges.

Komaroff, A.; Black, W.; Flatley, M.; Knapp, R.; Reiffen, B.; Sherman, H. February 7, 1974. Protocols for Physician Assistants. *New England Journal of Medicine* 290, no. 6:307–312.

Kramer, M. May 1974. *Reality Shock—Why Nurses Leave Nursing.* St. Louis, Missouri. Mosby.

Lawrence, D. 1974. Response to a Paper by Dr. Charles E. Lewis on "Training the New Health Practitioner." *Proceedings of The Institute on Primary Care.* October 6–8, 1974. Washington, D.C.: Association of American Medical Colleges.

Levy, B.; Wilkinson, F.; Marine, W. January 1, 1971. Reducing Neonatal Mortality Rate with Nurse-Midwives. *American Journal of Obstetrics and Gynecology* 109, no. 1:51–58.

Lewis, C. 1974. Training the New Health Practitioner. *Proceedings of The Institute on Primary Care.* October 6–8, 1974. Washington, D.C.: Association of American Medical Colleges.

Lewis, C.; Lorimer, A.; Lindeman, C.; Palmer, B.; Lewis, M. June 1974. An Evaluation of the Impact of School Nurse Practitioners. *Journal of School Health* 44, no. 6:331–335.

Lippard, V.; Purcell, E. eds. 1973. *Intermediate-Level Health Practitioners.* New York: Josiah Macy Jr. Foundation.

McDermott, W. November 1974. General Medical Care—Identification and Analysis of Alternative Approaches. *Johns Hopkins Medical Journal* 135, no. 5:292–321.

Machotka, P.; Ott, J. E.; Moon, J. B.; Silver, H. K. February 1973. Competence of Child Health Associates I. Comparison of their Basic Science and Clinical Knowledge with that of Medical Students and Pediatric Residents. *American Journal of Diseases of Children* 125:199–203. See also, Fall 1973. *The P.A. Journal—A Journal for New Health Practitioners* 3, no. 4:36–41.

Mahoney, M. 1973. The Future Role of Physician Assistants and Nurse Practitioners. *National Health Services: Their Impact on Medical Education and Their Role in Prevention,* Eds. Bowers, J. and Purcell, E. New York: Josiah Macy, Jr. Foundation.

Miike, L. March 1974. Institutional Licensure: An Experimental Model, Not a Solution. *Medical Care* 12, no. 3:214–220.

National Board of Medical Examiners. June 1973. *Evaluation in The Continuum of Medical Education. Report of the Committee on Goals and Priorities of the National Board of Medical Examiners.* Philadelphia: National Board of Medical Examiners.

National Council of MEDEX Programs. 1974. A Progress Report on MEDEX Programs in the United States. Mimeographed. University of Washington MEDEX Program.

Nelson, E.; Jacobs, A.; Nelson, J. Fall 1974. A Change in the Characteristics of MEDEX Applicants and Trainees. *The P.A. Journal—A Journal for New Health Practitioners* 4, no. 3:54–64.

Newhouse, P., Phelps, C. E., Schwartz, W. B. June 13, 1974. Policy Options and the Impact of National Health Insurance. *New England Journal of Medicine* 290, no. 24:1345–59.

Ornstein, R. E. 1972. *The Psychology of Consciousness.* San Francisco: W. H. Freeman and Company.

Peterson, M. 1974. Response to a Paper by Dr. David A. Kindig on "Primary Health Care Teams: Issues for Team Delivery and Interdisciplinary Education." *Proceedings of The Institute on Primary Care.* October 6–8, 1974. Washington, D.C.: Association of American Medical Colleges.

Pluckhan, M. 1972. Professional Territoriality: A Problem Affecting the Delivery of Health Care. *Nursing Forum* XI:3. See also, Summer 1974. *The P.A. Journal—A Journal for New Health Practitioners* 4, no. 2:41–45.

Pondy, L.; Jones, L.; Braun, J. 1973. Utilization and Productivity of the Duke Physician's Associate. *Socio-Economics Planning Sciences* 7:327–352.

Proceedings of The First National Conference on New Health Practitioners. Winter–Spring 1974. *The P.A. Journal—A Journal for New Health Practitioners* 4, no. 1:11–65.

Remen, N. 1975. *The Masculine Principle, The Feminine Principle and Humanistic Medicine.* San Francisco: Institute for the Study of Humanistic Medicine.

Rogers, D. December 1971. The Unity of Health: Reasonable Quest or Impossible Dream? *Journal of Medical Education* 46, no. 12:1047–1056.

Rogers, D. June 28, 1973. Shattuck Lecture—The American Health-Care Scene. Views from a Foundation Perspective. *New England Journal of Medicine* 288:1377–1383.

Ross, S. May 1973. The Clinical Nurse Practitioner in Ambulatory Care Service. *Bulletin of the New York Academy of Medicine* 49, no. 5:393–402.

Rubin, I.; Beckhard, R. July 1972. Factors Influencing the Effectiveness of Health Teams. *Milbank Memorial Fund Quarterly* p. 1:317–335.

Runyan, J. August 1972. The Public Health Nurse as a Practitioner in Chronic Disease Care. *Southern Medicine* 60, no. 4:15–19.

Runyan, J. 1975. *Primary Care Guide.* New York: Harper and Row.

Runyan, J. January 20, 1975. The Memphis Chronic Disease Program, Comparisons in Outcome and the Nurse's Extended Role. *JAMA* 231, no. 3:264–267.

Sackett, D. L.; Spitzer, W. O.; Gent, M.; Roberts, R. S. February 1974. The Burlington Randomized Trial of the Nurse Practitioner: Health Outcomes of Patients. *Annals of Internal Medicine* 80, no. 2:137–142. See also, Fall 1974. *The P.A. Journal—A Journal for New Health Practitioners* 4, no. 3:37–43.

Sadler, A. September 1974. The New Health Practitioner in Primary Care. *Journal of Medical Education* 49:845–848. See also, Summer 1974. *The P.A. Journal—A Journal for New Health Practitioners* 4, no. 2:35–37.

Sadler, A. 1974. Education of New Health Practitioners: Problems and Issues. *Proceedings of The Institute on Primary Care.* October 6–8, 1974. Washington, D.C.: Association of American Medical Colleges.

Scheffler, R.; Stinson, O. April 1973. Physician's Assistants: A Report on Earnings. *The P.A. Journal—A Journal for New Health Practitioners* 3, no. 2:11–18.

Schroeder, S.; Werner, S.; Piemme, T. September 1974. Primary Care in the Academic Medical Centers: A Report of a Survey by the AAMC. *Journal of Medical Education* 49:823–833.

Sherman, H.; Komaroff, A. August 1974. *Progress Report: Ambulatory Care Project 1969–1974.* Boston: Lincoln Laboratory, Massachusetts Institute of Technology and Beth Israel Hospital, Harvard Medical School.

Silver, H. April 1974. New Health Professionals for Primary Ambulatory Care. *Hospital Practice* 9, no. 4:91–98.

Sims, N.; Seidel, H.; Cooke, R. July 1971. A Structured Approach to the Use of Physician Extenders in Well-Child Evaluations. *The Journal of Pediatrics* 79, no. 1:151–163.

Smith, R. A. April 1974. Towards Solving the "Great Training Robbery." *Pharos* 37, no. 2:47–52.

Sox, H.; Sox, C.; Tompkins, R. April 19, 1973. The Training of Physician's Assistants: The Use of the Clinical Algorithm System for Patient Care, Audit of Performance and Education. *New England Journal of Medicine* 288:818–24. See also, Summer 1973. *The P.A. Journal—A Journal for New Health Practitioners* 3, no. 3:6–14.

Spitzer, W. O. 1974. Response to a Paper by Dr. David A. Kindig on "Primary Health Care Teams: Issues for Team Delivery and Interdisciplinary Education." *Proceedings of The Institute on Primary Care.* October 6–8, 1974. Washington, D.C.: Association of American Medical Colleges.

Spitzer, W. O.; Sackett, D. L. et al. January 31, 1974. The Burlington Randomized Trial of the Nurse Practitioner. *New England Journal of Medicine* 290, no. 5:251–256.

Storms, D. 1974. *Training of the Nurse Practitioner: A Clinical and Statistical Analysis.* New Haven: Connecticut Health Services Research Series No. 4.

Sultz, H. A. 1975. Role Preparation and Expectations of Nurses in Extended Roles. Paper presented at Nurse Practitioner World Conference II. April 30—May 2, 1975, at Hartford, Connecticut.

Tichy, M. 1974. *Health Care Teams—An Annotated Bibliography.* New York: Praeger Publishers.

Todd, M. October 30, 1972. National Certification of Physician's Assistants by Uniform Examinations. *JAMA* 222, no. 5:563–566.

Todd, M. Winter–Spring 1974. The Physician's Assistant: In Perspective. *The P.A. Journal—A Journal for New Health Practitioners* 4, no. 1:5–7.

Torrey, E.; Smith, D.; Wise, H. January 1973. The Family Health Worker Revisited: A Five-Year Follow-up. *American Journal of Public Health* 63, no. 1:71–74.

U.S. Department of Health, Education and Welfare. 1973. *Report of the Secretary's Commission on Medical Malpractice.* HEW pub. no. (OS) 73–88. Washington, D.C.: U.S. Government Printing Office.

U.S. Department of Health, Education and Welfare. 1973. *Report of the Secretary's Commission on Medical Malpractice, Appendix: Reports,*

Studies and Analyses. HEW pub. no. (OS) 73–89. Washington, D.C.: U.S. Government Printing Office.

White, K. L.; Williams, T. F.; Greenberg, B. G. November 2, 1961. The Ecology of Medical Care. New England Journal of Medicine 265, no. 19:885–892.

Wise, H.; Beckhard, R.; Rubin, I.; Kyte, A. 1974. Making Health Teams Work. Cambridge, Mass.: Ballinger Publishing Company.

World Health Organization. 1974. The Medical Assistant—An Intermediate Level of Health Care Personnel. June 5–7, 1973. Bethesda, Md.

Zeckhauser, R.; Eliastam, M. Winter 1974. Productivity Potential of the Physician Assistant. Journal of Human Resources 9:95–116.

Appendixes

PA and Nurse Practitioner Programs

This list of PA programs was compiled from the AMA "Accredited Educational Programs to the Assistant to the Primary Care Physician," December 1974, and from Association of Physician Assistant Programs, *Profile 1975–76*, pp. 21–29.

For further information contact:

American Medical Association
Department of Health Manpower
535 North Dearborn Street
Chicago, Illinois 60610

or

Association of Physician Assistant Programs
National Office
The Gelman Building, Suite 210
2120 L Street, N.W.
Washington, D.C. 20037

State / Program	Entrance Requirements	Length of Program	Award	Class Size
ALABAMA University of Alabama Physician's Assistant Program 1919 Seventh Avenue South University Station Birmingham, AL 35233	2 years health experience; 2 years college or equivalent	24 months	B.S. and certificate	25
University of Alabama Surgeon's Assistant Program Birmingham, AL 35233		23 months	B.S. and certificate	10
ARIZONA Phoenix Indian Medical Center Community Health Medic Program 4212 North Sixteenth Street Phoenix, AZ 85016	3 years patient care experience; High school diploma or equivalent	24 months	Certificate and A.S. degree	10
CALIFORNIA University of California—Davis Family Nurse Practitioner/ Physician's Assistant Program Department of Family Practice Davis, CA 95616	2 years ambulatory care experience; that applicant be a registered nurse (2, 3, or 4 year)	18 months	M.H.S. or certificate	75
UCLA & Charles R. Drew Post- Graduate Medical School PA/MEDEX Program	3 years health experience; 30 semester units of college credit	15 months	Certificate and A.S. degree	36

Institution / Address	Prerequisites	Duration	Credential	No.
1620 East 119th Street Los Angeles, CA 90002				
COLORADO University of Colorado Medical Center Child Health Associate Program 4200 East Ninth Avenue Denver, CO 80220	2 years college or equivalent	36 months	B.S., M.S., certificate	14
CONNECTICUT Yale University School of Medicine Physician's Associate Program 382 Congress Avenue New Haven, CT 06510	Baccalaureate degree; strongly recommend substantial direct patient care experience; SAT scores	24 months	Certificate	21
DISTRICT OF COLUMBIA George Washington University School of Medicine Physician's Assistant Program 1331 H Street, N.W. Washington, D.C. 20037	One year patient care experience; high school diploma or equivalent; post-high school medical training or college education; preference for health experience; ex-military corpsman with a minimum of 14 weeks of medical training	24 months	Certificate and B.S. degree	40
Howard University College of Medicine PA/MEDEX Program 520 W Street, N.W. Washington, D.C. 20037	3 years patient care experience; 2 years college or equivalent	15 months	Certificate	24

State Program	Entrance Requirements	Length of Program	Award	Class Size
FLORIDA Santa Fe Community College Physician's Assistant Program 4350 S.W. Thirteenth Street P.O. Box 1550, Room 13 Gainesville, FL 32601	High school diploma or equivalent; 2 years patient care experience or a baccalaureate degree	24 months	A.S. degree and certificate	35
GEORGIA Emory University Physician's Associate Program Woodruff Memorial Building Atlanta, GA 30322	SAT or ACT scores; high school diploma or equivalent; prefer patient experience	24–27 mos.	A.M. or B.M.Sc.	40
Medical College of Georgia Physician's Assistant Program Fifteenth Street Augusta, GA 30902	3 years patient care experience; 2 years college or equivalent	24 months	B.S. and certificate	24
INDIANA Indiana University School of Medicine Physician's Assistant Program 960 Locke Street Indianapolis, IN 46805	1 year patient care experience; 1 year college or equivalent	24 months	Certificate	20

IOWA

University of Iowa College of Medicine
Physician's Assistant Program
Dean's Office
Iowa City, IA 52240

Program	Prerequisites	Length	Credential	No.
University of Iowa College of Medicine, Physician's Assistant Program, Dean's Office, Iowa City, IA 52240	2 years college or equivalent; prefer health experience	24 months	B.S. and certificate	30

KANSAS

Wichita State University
Physician's Assistant Program
1845 Fairmont
Wichita, Kansas 67208

Wichita State University, Physician's Assistant Program, 1845 Fairmont, Wichita, Kansas 67208	3 years patient care experience or a baccalaureate degree	24 months	Certificate	25

KENTUCKY

The University of Kentucky
Clinical Associate Program
Medical Center Annex #1, Room 15
Lexington, KY 40506

The University of Kentucky, Clinical Associate Program, Medical Center Annex #1, Room 15, Lexington, KY 40506	High school diploma or equivalent; 2 years in medicine	22 months	Certificate	10

MARYLAND

Essex Community College
Physician's Assistant Program
Baltimore County, MD 21236

Essex Community College, Physician's Assistant Program, Baltimore County, MD 21236	High school diploma or equivalent	24 months	A.A. degree	30

Johns Hopkins University
School of Health Services
Health Associate Program
624 North Broadway
Baltimore, MD 21205

Johns Hopkins University, School of Health Services, Health Associate Program, 624 North Broadway, Baltimore, MD 21205	2 years college or equivalent	21 months	B.A. degree	36

State	Program	Entrance Requirements	Length of Program	Award	Class Size
MASSACHUSETTS	Northeastern University Physician's Assistant Program 360 Huntington Avenue Boston, MA 02115	High school diploma or equivalent; post-high school training or college; 1–2 years patient care experience	18 months	Certificate	25
MICHIGAN	Mercy College of Detroit Physician's Assistant Program 8200 West Outer Drive Detroit, MI 48219	High school diploma or equivalent; post-high school training or education; 2 years health or patient care experience	24 months	B.S. degree	25
	Western Michigan University Physician's Assistant Program The Graduate College Kalamazoo, MI 49001	2 years college or equivalent	24 months	B.S. in Medicine	42
MISSOURI	St. Louis University School of Nursing and Allied Health Professions Physician's Assistant Program 1401 South Garland Boulevard St. Louis, MO 63104	2 years patient care experience; 2 years college or equivalent; ex-military corpsman, minimum 14 weeks medical training	24 months	Certificate	16

Program	Prerequisites	Length	Degree	
NEBRASKA University of Nebraska Medical Center Physician's Assistant Program 42nd and Dewey Avenue Omaha, NB 68105	40 semester hours of college	24 months	B.S. degree	15
NEW MEXICO Gallup Indian Medical Center Community Health Medic Program P.O. Box 1337, Drawer L Gallup, NM 87301	3 years patient care experience; high school diploma or equivalent	24 months	A.S. (by the University of New Mexico) and certificate	15
NEW YORK Albany Medical College/Hudson Valley Community College Physician's Associate Program 47 New Scotland Avenue Albany, NY 12208	High school diploma or equivalent; ACT and/or SAT scores; 1 year patient care experience	24 months	A.A.S. degree and certificate	36
Antioch College/Harlem Hospital Physician's Associate Program 530 Lenox Avenue New York City, NY 10037	High school diploma or equivalent; 2 years patient care experience; ex-military corpsman 14 weeks medical training	24 months	B.S. degree	20
The Brooklyn Hospital Physician's Associate Program 121 Dekalb Avenue Brooklyn, NY 11201	High school diploma or equivalent; 1 year patient care experience; ACT or SAT scores	36 months	B.S. degree	44

State	Program	Entrance Requirements	Length of Program	Award	Class Size
	State University of New York Physician's Associate Program School of Allied Health Stony Brook, NY 11790	High school diploma or equivalent; 1 year patient care experience	24 months	B.S. degree and certificate	30
	Touro College Physician's Associate Program 30 West 44th Street New York, NY 10036	High school diploma or equivalent; 2 years college or equivalent; prefer health experience	24 months	B.S. degree	100
	U.S. Public Health Service Hospital Physician's Assistant Program Bay and Vanderbilt Streets Staten Island, NY 10304	High school diploma or equivalent; 3 years medical experience	24 months	Certificate	40
NORTH CAROLINA	Bowman Gray School of Medicine of Wake Forest University Physician's Assistant Program 300 South Hawthorne Road Winston-Salem, NC 27103	High school diploma or equivalent; 2 years experience as a medical corpsman or 2 years college and/or patient care experience	24 months	Certificate and/or degree	40
	Duke University School of Medicine Physician's Associate Program Duke University Medical Center Durham, NC 27710	High school diploma or equivalent; 1 year patient care experience (for baccalaureate degree, 2 years college also required)	24 months	B.H.S. and certificate	40

Program	Prerequisites	Length	Credential	Enrollment
NORTH DAKOTA University of North Dakota MEDEX Program University Station Grand Forks, ND 58201	High school diploma or equivalent; 3 years medical experience; prefer military medical corpsman or RN	12 months	Certificate	20
OHIO Cincinnati Technical College Physician's Assistant Program 3420 Central Parkway Cincinnati, OH 45223	High school diploma or equivalent; prefer health experience	24 months	Certificate	20
Cuyahoga Community College Physician's Assistant Program 2214 East Fourteenth Street Cleveland, OH 44115	High school diploma or equivalent	21 months	A.S. degree	25
Kettering College of Medical Arts Physician's Assistant Program Kettering, OH		23 months	A.S. degree	15
OKLAHOMA University of Oklahoma Health Sciences Center Physician's Associate Program 721 N.E. Fourteenth P.O. Box 26901 Oklahoma City, OK 73190	2 years health experience; 2 years college or equivalent	24 months	B.H. degree	30

State	Program	Entrance Requirements	Length of Program	Award	Class Size
PENNSYLVANIA	Hahnemann Medical College and Hospital Physician's Assistant Program 230 North Broad Street Philadelphia, PA 19102	High school diploma or equivalent	21 months	A.S. degree	30
	The Pennsylvania State University MEDEX Program 212 J. Orvis Keller Building University Park, PA 19102 (Program site is in Hershey, PA)	High school diploma or equivalent; 2 years direct clinical care experience; U.S. citizen; 14 weeks medical training or equivalent	15 months	Certificate	25
SOUTH CAROLINA	Medical University of South Carolina MEDEX Program 80 Barre Street Charleston, SC 29401	High school diploma or equivalent; 3 years patient care experience; ex-military corpsman and 14 weeks medical training	12 months	Certificate	25
TEXAS	Baylor College of Medicine Physician's Assistant Program Houston, TX 77025	2 years college or equivalent; 2 years health experience	24 months	B.S. degree and certificate	40
	University of Texas Health Science Center at Dallas Physician's Assistant Program	2 years college or equivalent	24 months	B.S. degree	24

5323 Harry Hines Boulevard
Dallas, TX 75235

University of Texas Medical Branch at Galveston Physician's Assistant Program Galveston, TX 77550	2 years college or equivalent	26 months	B.S. degree and certificate	20
United States Air Force School of Health Care Sciences Physician's Assistant Program Sheppard Air Force Base Wichita Falls, TX 76311	High school diploma or equivalent; 1 year patient care experience; medical service airman with 3 years service	24 months	B.S. degree	65
U.S. Army Academy of Health Sciences Physician's Assistant Program Fort Sam Houston San Antonio, TX 76311	High school diploma or equivalent; Army GT score of 100; 3 years clinical experience	24 months	A.S. degree	60
UTAH University of Utah MEDEX Program Salt Lake City, UT 84112	Extensive previous training and experience	12 months	Certificate	15
WASHINGTON University of Washington/Washington State Medical Society MEDEX-Northwest Program 444 North East Ravenna Boulevard Seattle, WA 98115	3 years medical experience and/or education; 14 weeks medical training as military corpsman	12 months	Certificate	15

State Program	Entrance Requirements	Length of Program	Award	Class Size
WEST VIRGINIA Alderson-Broaddus College Physician's Assistant Program Division of Professional Studies Philippi, WV 36416	High school diploma or equivalent	42 months	B.S. degree	40
WISCONSIN Marshfield Clinic Foundation Physician's Assistant Program 510 North St. Joseph Avenue Marshfield, WI 54449	High school diploma or equivalent; 3 years prior pertinent experience or registered nurse diploma	24 months	Certificate	20

This list of nurse practitioner programs has been compiled from HEW publication no. (NIH) 74–31, entitled Preparing Registered Nurses for Expanded Roles. It was prepared jointly by:

The American Nurses' Association, Inc.
2420 Pershing Road
Kansas City, Missouri 64108

and

The U.S. Department of Health, Education and Welfare
Public Health Service
Health Resources Administration
Bureau of Health Resources Development
Division of Manpower Intelligence
9000 Rockville Pike
Bethesda, Maryland 20014

NOTE: Although comprehensive and representative, this is not a complete listing of all programs to prepare nurses for expanded roles.

I.   Programs that Award a Certificate (arranged alphabetically by state, program, and city)

State Program (Nurse Specialty Title) Address	Entrance Requirements	Length of Program
ALABAMA *Pediatric Nurse Practitioner* University of Alabama School of Nursing Box 1 1919 Seventh Avenue South Birmingham 35233	RN licensure in Alabama; experience in nursing of children; liability insurance	6 months
ARIZONA *Family Nurse Practitioner* University of Arizona College of Nursing and Medicine Tucson 85721	Practicing RN from accredited school; 2 years experience as graduate nurse; meet requirements of University of Arizona; ACT test scores	12 months
Pediatric Nurse Associate Good Samaritan Hospital P.O. Box 2989 1033 East Mcdowell Road Phoenix 85062	Graduate of an accredited school of nursing; RN licensure; previous experience in pediatrics; commitment from employer or sponsor	16 weeks
ARKANSAS *Pediatric Nurse Practitioner* University of Arkansas School of Medicine	RN licensure	9 months

Department of Pediatrics
4301 West Markham Street
Little Rock 72205

CALIFORNIA
Child Nurse Associate
University of California
School of Nursing
Second and Parnassus
San Francisco 94122

RN licensure

2 quarters

Family Nurse Practitioner
University of California
School of Medicine
Department of Family Practice
Davis 95616

RN licensure; 2 years community
nursing experience

12 months

Family Nurse Practitioner
University of California
Center for Health Sciences
10833 Le Conte Avenue
Los Angeles 90024

RN licensure; sponsored

1 year

Maternal Nurse Associate
University of California
School of Nursing
Second and Parnarssus
San Francisco 94122

RN licensure; state resident

6 months

State Program *(Nurse Specialty Title)*	Address	Entrance Requirements	Length of Program
Pediatric Nurse Associate Loma Linda University Loma Linda 92354		RN licensure in California; public health certificate; Baccalaureate in nursing; SAT and California Psychology Inventory	6 months
Pediatric Nurse Practitioner University of California School of Medicine Department of Pediatrics 225 West Dickerson Street San Diego 92103		RN licensure in California; public health nurse and/or 1 year in pediatric nursing; state resident	6 months
School Nurse Specialist University of Southern California School of Medicine 1200 North State Street Los Angeles 90033		RN licensure; degree from college	12 months
COLORADO *Adult Health Care Practitioner* University of Colorado School of Nursing 4200 East 9th Avenue Denver 80220		RN licensure; B.S.; 1 year of nursing experience employment; letter of commitment from physician to serve as preceptor	2½ months

Pediatric Nurse Practitioner
University of Colorado
School of Nursing
4200 East 9th Avenue
Denver 80220

RN licensure; B.S. in nursing;
commitment of employment

4 months

Rural Health Care Nurse
University of Colorado
School of Nursing
4200 East 9th Avenue
Denver 80220

RN licensure; diploma or certificate
from accredited school of nursing

3 weeks

School Nurse Practitioner
University of Colorado Medical Center
4200 East 9th Avenue
Denver 80220

RN licensure

12 months

CONNECTICUT
Pediatric Nurse Associate
University of Connecticut
School of Medicine and Nursing
2 Holcomb Street
Hartford 06112

RN licensure; graduate from
NLN accredited
B.A. Nursing Program

4 months

DISTRICT OF COLUMBIA
Nurse-Midwife
Georgetown University
School of Nursing
3700 Reservoir Road, N.W.
Washington 10007

RN licensure; 1 year experience
in obstetrics, preferably in labor
and delivery

9 months

State Program (Nurse Specialty Title)	Address	Entrance Requirements	Length of Program
FLORIDA			
Pediatric Nurse Practitioner	Palm Beach Junior College School of Nursing 4200 Congress Avenue West Palm Beach 33401	RN licensure; experience in pediatric nursing	12 months
ILLINOIS			
Medical Nurse Associate	Rush Presbyterian/ St. Luke's Medical Center 1753 West Congress Parkway Chicago 60612	RN licensure; graduate from an accredited school of nursing; pediatric sponsor	6 months
Nurse-Midwife	University of Illinois College of Nursing Department of Maternal-Child Nursing P.O. Box 6998 Chicago 60680	RN licensure; B.S. in nursing	5 quarters
Pediatric Nurse Associate	Rush Presbyterian/ St. Luke's Medical Center 1753 West Congress Parkway Chicago 60612	RN licensure; graduate from an accredited school of nursing	6 months

INDIANA *Family Nurse Practitioner* Regenstreif Institute for Health Care Marion County General Hospital 960 Locke Street Indianapolis 46202	RN licensure	1 year
Pediatric Nurse Associate Indiana University School of Nursing 1800 North Capital Avenue Indianapolis 46202	RN licensure; 2 years experience, preferably ambulatory pediatrics; commitment of employment	4 months
IOWA *Pediatric Nurse Practitioner* University of Iowa College of Nursing and Medicine Iowa City 52242	RN licensure; experience in ambulatory pediatrics; commitment of employment	4 months
KENTUCKY *Midwife and Family Nurse Practitioner* Frontier Nursing Service, Inc. Wendover 41775	RN—eligible for licensure in Kentucky; 1 year experience in nursing	12 months (16 months with mid- wifery
MAINE *Family Nurse Associate* University of Maine at Portland-Gorham 112 Vaughn Street Portland 04102	RN licensure in Maine; sponsored by and returned to an agency, institution, or doctor's office; state resident; commitment of employment	4 months

State Program (Nurse Specialty Title) Address	Entrance Requirements	Length of Program
Family Nurse Practitioner Medical Care Development, Inc. 295 Walter Street Augusta 04330	Consult institution	Consult institution
Pediatric Nurse Associate University of Maine 96 Falmouth Street Portland 04103	RN licensure; 1 year experience in public health or pediatric nursing	4 months
MARYLAND *Pediatric Nurse Practitioner* Johns Hopkins University School of Health Sciences 500 North Broadway Baltimore 21205	RN licensure; diploma; 2 years experience in pediatrics ambulatory care; commitment of employment	4 months
Primary Care Nurse Practitioner University of Maryland School of Nursing 655 West Hombard Street Baltimore 21201	RN licensure; prefer 2-3 years of ambulatory clinical experience	5 months

MASSACHUSETTS

Pediatric Nurse Associate
Northeastern University
College of Nursing
11 Leon Street
Boston 02115

RN licensure; diploma; baccalaureate
degree; experience in ambulatory setting;
commitment of employment

4 months

MICHIGAN

Pediatric Nurse Practitioner
University of Michigan
School of Nursing
1355 Catherine Street
Ann Arbor 48104

RN from an accredited school;
1 year experience (includes working
with children); commitment of
employment

8 months

Pediatric Nurse Practitioner
Children's Hospital of Michigan
3901 Beaubien
Detroit 48201

RN licensure; nursing degree;
postgraduate experience

4 months

MINNESOTA

Adult Health Associate
University of Minnesota
School of Public Health
1325 Mayo Memorial Building
Minneapolis 55455

RN licensure

6 months

Adult Nurse Associate
School of Public Health
University of Minnesota
1325 Mayo Memorial Building
Minneapolis 55455

RN licensure; diploma from school
of nursing; 2 years nursing experience;
California Psychology inventory;
physician mentor

5 months

State Program (Nurse Specialty Title)	Address	Entrance Requirements	Length of Program
Ambulatory Child Health Care Nurse *(postbaccalaureate training)* University of Minnesota School of Public Health 1325 Mayo Memorial Building Minneapolis 55455		RN licensure; college degree in nursing; 2 years experience professional nursing; California personality inventory, MMPI; strong vocational interest	9 months
Pediatric Nurse Associate Health Related Science Programs Mayo Foundation 200 First Street, S.W. Rochester 55901		RN licensure; diploma	6 months
MISSISSIPPI *Family Planning Nurse Practitioner* University of Mississippi Medical Center Department of Obstetrics-Gynetrics 2500 North State Street Jackson 39216		RN licensure; commitment of employment	2 months
Nurse-Midwife University of Mississippi Medical Center Department of Obstetrics-Gynetrics 2500 North State Street Jackson 39216		RN licensure; baccalaureate; 1 year experience nursing; GRE, MMIP	12 months

MISSOURI

Family Nurse Practitioner University of Missouri School of Medicine Columbia 65201	Consult institution	Consult institution
Nurse-Midwife St. Louis University School of Nursing and Allied Health Profession 1401 South Grand Boulevard St. Louis 63104	Consult institution	Consult institution
Pediatric Nurse Associate The Children's Mercy Hospital 24th at Gillham Road Kansas City 64108	RN licensure; baccalaureate; nursing experience in pediatrics	12 months
Pediatric Nurse Practitioner Cardinal Glennon Memorial Hospital 1465 Brand Boulevard St. Louis 63130	RN licensure; commitment of employment	8 months
Pediatric Nurse Practitioner Washington University School of Medicine 4456 Scott Avenue St. Louis 63110	RN licensure; experience in pediatric nursing	8½ months

State Program (Nurse Specialty Title)	Address	Entrance Requirements	Length of Program
MONTANA *Family Health Practitioner*	Montana State University School of Nursing Bozeman 59715	RN licensure; commitment from physician to serve as preceptor	9 months
NEW JERSEY *Pediatric Nurse Associate*	Seton Hall University School of Nursing South Orange 07079	RN licensure; B.S.; child nursing experience	4 months
Pediatric Nurse Practitioner	Rutgers College of Nursing and the College of Medicine and Dentistry of New Jersey P.O. Box 101 Piscataway 08854	RN licensure; baccalaureate degree	10 months
NEW YORK *Family Nurse Practitioner*	Cornell University New York Hospital School of Nursing 1320 York Avenue New York 10021	RN licensure; sponsored	1 year

Medical Nurse Practitioner
University of Rochester
School of Nursing
260 Crittenden Blvd.
Rochester 14642

RN licensure; degree or diploma in nursing; inpatient or ambulatory nursing experience; evidence of employment in a nurse practitioner role, evidence of collaboration with a physician who will cooperate in the training program

8 months

Nurse-Midwife
State University of New York
College of Health Related Professions
Downstate Medical Center
450 Clarkson Avenue
Brooklyn 11203

RN licensure in New York; 1 year professional nursing experience; SAT

8 months

Nurse-Midwife (postmaster's program)
State University of New York
College of Health Related Professions
450 Clarkson Avenue
Brooklyn 11203

RN licensure in New York; 1 year experience as nurse or teacher; GRE

6 months

Pediatric Nurse Associate
State University of New York
School of Nursing
3435 Main Street
Buffalo 14214

RN licensure in New York; experience in pediatric or public health nursing; commitment of employment

4 months

State Program (Nurse Specialty Title)	Address	Entrance Requirements	Length of Program
Pediatric Nurse Associate	Cornell University New York Hospital School of Nursing 1320 York Avenue New York 10021	RN licensure in New York; employed as public health nurse by New York City Health Department; NLN prenursing and guidance examination	12 months
Pediatric Nurse Practitioner	Bronx Municipal Hospital Center Pelham Parkway and Eastchester Road Bronx 10461	RN licensure; 1 year nursing experience, preferably in pediatrics	4 months
Pediatric Nurse Practitioner	University of Rochester School of Nursing 260 Crittenden Boulevard Rochester 14620	RN licensure; evidence of employment in a nurse practitioner role; employment in pediatrics	4 months
NORTH CAROLINA *Family Nurse Practitioner*	University of North Carolina School of Nursing Chapel Hill 27514	RN licensure; state resident	12 months
NORTH DAKOTA *Family Nurse Practitioner*	University of North Dakota Department of Commercial Medicine 1600 University Avenue	RN licensure; degree or diploma	12 months

1600 University Avenue
Grand Forks 58201

OHIO

Family Nurse Practitioner
Case Western Reserve University
Francis Payne Bolton School
of Nursing
2121 Arlington Road
Cleveland 44106

RN licensure

4 months

Pediatric Nurse Associate
Good Samaritan Hospital
Department of Pediatrics
3217 Clifton Avenue
Cincinnati 45220

RN licensure; degree or diploma
from NLN approved school;
employment in ambulatory setting

4 months

OKLAHOMA

Pediatric–School Nurse Associate
Tulsa City—County Health Department
4616 East 15th Street
Tulsa 74112

RN licensure; pediatric sponsor
in Oklahoma

2½ months

PENNSYLVANIA

Pediatric Nurse Practitioner
University of Pittsburgh
School of Medicine and Nursing
Pittsburgh 15213

RN licensure; baccalaureate degree
in nursing; 2 years experience in
clinical pediatrics

10 months

State / Program (Nurse Specialty Title)	Address	Entrance Requirements	Length of Program
PUERTO RICO			
Nurse-Midwife	University District Hospital School of Nurse-Midwifery Caparra Heights 00920	RN licensure; 2 years experience in maternity care; commitment of employment	6 months
TENNESSEE			
Family Nurse Practitioner	Vanderbilt University School of Nursing 21st Avenue South Nashville 37203	RN licensure; 2 years experience	12 months
Pediatric Nurse Associate	University of Tennessee College of Nursing 879 Madison Avenue Memphis 38103	RN licensure; BA degree in nursing	20 weeks
Pediatric Nurse Practitioner	Meharry Medical College 1005 18th Avenue North Nashville 37208	RN licensure; graduate from NLN approved school; 2 years experience in nursing	9 months

TEXAS		
Clinical Specialist (in care of the thermally injured)		
University of Texas Southwestern Medical School Department of Surgery 5323 Harry Hines Boulevard Dallas 75223	RN licensed; B.S. in nursing	2 years
Pediatric Nurse Practitioner		
University of Texas School of Nursing Brackenridge Hall Galveston 77550	RN licensure; experience in ambulatory child health care setting	4 months
Pediatric Nurse Practitioner		
USAF Medical Center Wilford Hall Lackland AFB San Antonio 78236	RN licensure; 2 years experience as military RN (1 year in pediatrics); must be on active duty with U.S. Air Force	21 weeks
VIRGINIA		
Family Nurse Practitioner		
Virginia Commonwealth University School of Nursing 1220 East Broad Street Richmond 23219	RN licensed to practice in Virginia; 1 year experience of primary care; state resident; actively practiced nursing within last 5 years or has taken refresher course; has position to fill as nurse practitioner in Virginia	9–12 months

State Program (Nurse Specialty Title)	Address	Entrance Requirements	Length of Program
Nurse Practitioner (adult and adolescent care)	University of Virginia School of Medicine Charlottesville 22901	RN licensure; diploma; 3 years experience	5 months
Pediatric Nurse Clinician	University of Virginia School of Nursing McLeod Building Charlottesville 22901	RN licensure; 1-2 years pediatric nursing practice	4 months
WASHINGTON *Pediatric Nurse Practitioner*	University of Washington School of Nursing Health Sciences Building Seattle 98105	RN licensure; work experience; physician sponsor	3 months
WEST VIRGINIA *Pediatric Nurse Associate*	West Virginia University Medical Center School of Nursing Morgantown 26505	RN licensure; diploma; experience in pediatric nursing	10 months

WISCONSIN

Nurse Associate (physician team)
University of Wisconsin—Extension
Lake Street
Madison 53706

RN licensure in Wisconsin or adjacent state; 1 year experience as nurse; must be enrolled with a pediatrician, general practitioner, or family practitioner — 6½ months

---

II. Programs that Award a Master's Degree in Nursing (arranged alphabetically by state and city)

State Address	Area of Concentration (Occupational Title)	Entrance Requirements	Length of Program
ALABAMA University of Alabama School of Nursing Box 1, 1919 Seventh Avenue, South Birmingham 35233	Cardiovascular N.C. Community Health N.P. Maternal N.P. Medical-Surgical N.P. Pediatric N.P. Psychiatric N.C. Rehabilitation N.P.	B.S. in nursing RN licensure Miller Analogies Test	4 quarters
ARIZONA Arizona State University College of Nursing Tempe 85281	Community Health N.P. Community Mental Health Nurse Family-Child N.C. Medical-Surgical N.P. Psychiatric Nurse	B.S. in nursing RN licensure GRE	4 semesters

State / Address	Area of Concentration (Occupational Title)	Entrance Requirements	Length of Program
University of Arizona College of Nursing Tucson 85721	Community Health N.C. Maternal and Newborn N.C. Medical-Surgical N.C. Pediatric N.C. Psychiatric-Mental Health N.C.	B.S. in nursing RN licensure GRE	12 months
CALIFORNIA California State College Department of Nursing 5151 State College Drive Los Angeles 90032	Adult N.S. Child N.S.	B.S. in nursing RN licensure GRE	4 quarters
Fresno State College Department of Nursing Fresno 93710	Curriculum being revised, consult institution	B.S. in nursing RN licensure GRE NLN comprehensive examination in clinical area selected by applicant	2 semesters and 1 summer session
Loma Linda University School of Nursing Loma Linda 92354	Community Health Nurse Maternal-Child Nurse Medical-Surgical Nurse Nurse-Midwife Psychiatric Nurse	B.S. in nursing RN licensure Miller Analogies Test, Dopplet Math	5 quarters

University of California School of Nursing 10833 Le Conte Avenue Los Angeles 90024	Community Mental Health Nurse Maternal-Child Nurse Medical-Surgical Nurse Obstetrical N.C. Pediatric N.P. Public Health Nurse School Nurse Psychiatric-Mental Health N.C.	B.S. in nursing RN licensure	5 or 6 quarters
University of California School of Nursing San Francisco 94122	Community Health N.C. Maternal-Child C.N.S. Medical-Surgical Nurse Psychiatric-Mental Health N.C.	B.S. in nursing RN licensure GRE	3 quarters
COLORADO University of Colorado School of Nursing 4200 Fast 9th Avenue Medical Center Denver 80220	Community Health N.C. Maternal-Child N.C. Medical-Surgical N.C. Psychiatric-Mental Health N.C.	B.S. in nursing RN licensure GRE	1 or 2 years
CONNECTICUT Yale University School of Nursing 38 South Street New Haven 06510	Family N.P. Pediatric C.S. Psychiatric C.S. Public Health C.S. Nurse-Midwife	Baccalaureate from an accredited college RN licensure GRE	4 semesters

State / Address	Area of Concentration (Occupational Title)	Entrance Requirements	Length of Program
DELAWARE University of Delaware College of Nursing Newark 19711	Community Health Specialist Maternal-Child N.C.	B.S. in nursing RN licensure GRE	2 academic years
DISTRICT OF COLUMBIA Catholic University of America School of Nursing 3800 Brookland Avenue, N.E. Washington 20017	Cardiovascular N.C. Community Health N.C. Maternal-Infant N.C. Medical-Surgical N.C. Psychiatric-Mental Health N.C.	B.S. in nursing RN licensure Miller Analogies Test	3–4 semesters
FLORIDA University of Florida J.H. Miller Health Center College of Nursing Gainesville 32601	Maternal-Child N.C. Medical-Surgical N.C. Pediatric N.C. Psychiatric-Mental Health N.C.	B.S. in nursing RN licensure GRE	4 quarters
GEORGIA Emory University Nell Hodgson Woodruff School of Nursing Atlanta 30322	Maternity N.C. Medical-Surgical N.C. Pediatric N.C. Psychiatric N.C. Public Health N.C.	B.S. in nursing RN licensure Plan A—NLN Graduate Nurse Examination	4 quarters

School	Major	Requirements	Length
HAWAII University of Hawaii School of Nursing 2528 The Mall Honolulu 96822	Medical-Surgical N.C. Psychiatric-Mental Health N.C.	B.S. in nursing RN licensure GRE	4 semesters
ILLINOIS Loyola University of Chicago School of Nursing 6525 North Sheridan Road Chicago 60626	Adult N.S.	B.S. in nursing RN licensure GRE	13½ months
Saint Xavier College School of Nursing 103rd and Central Park Avenue Chicago 60655	Psychiatric-Mental Health N.C.	B.S. in nursing RN licensure Miller Analogies Test	4 semesters
INDIANA Indiana University School of Nursing 1232 West Michigan Street Indianapolis 46202	Psychiatric-Mental Health C.S.	B.S. in nursing RN licensure GRE	4 semesters and 1 summer session
IOWA University of Iowa College of Nursing Iowa City 52240	Child N.S. Medical-Surgical N.C. Psychiatric-Mental Health N.C.	B.S. in nursing RN licensure GRE	3 semesters

State / Address	Area of Concentration (Occupational Title)	Entrance Requirements	Length of Program
MARYLAND University of Maryland School of Nursing 655 West Lombard Street Baltimore 21201	Community Health N.C. Maternal-Child N.C. Medical-Surgical N.C. Psychiatric-Child N.C. Psychiatric N.C.	B.S. in nursing RN licensure	3 or 4 semesters
Johns Hopkins University School of Hygiene and Public Health 615 North Wolfe Street Baltimore 21205	Nurse-Midwife	Consult institution	Consult institution
MASSACHUSETTS University of Massachusetts School of Nursing Amherst 01002	Medical-Surgical N.C. Psychiatric-Mental Health N.C.	B.S. in nursing GRE or Miller Analogies Test	2 academic years
Boston University School of Nursing 635 Commonwealth Avenue Boston 02215	Community Health N.C. Maternal-Child N.C. Medical-Surgical N.C. Psychiatric-Mental Health N.C. Rehabilitation N.C.	B.S. in nursing RN licensure Miller Analogies Test	3 semesters
Boston College School of Nursing 140 Commonwealth Avenue Chestnut Hill 02167	Community Health Nurse Maternity Distributive Care C.S. Medical-Surgical Nurse Pediatric Distributive Care C.S. Psychiatric-Mental Health N.C.	B.S. in nursing RN licensure GRE	2 years

MICHIGAN

University of Michigan
School of Nursing
1355 Catherine Street
Ann Arbor 48104

Medical-Surgical C.N.S.
Psychiatric C.N.S.

B.S. in nursing
RN licensure
Miller Analogies Test

2 academic
years

Wayne State University
College of Nursing
5557 Cass Avenue
Detroit 48202

Adult Psychiatry C.S.
Child N.C.S.
Health N.C.
Maternity N.C.S.
Medical-Surgical N.C.S.
Psychiatric N.C.S.

B.S. in nursing
RN licensure
GRE

6 quarters

MINNESOTA

University of Minnesota
School of Nursing
Minneapolis 55455

Adult Health N.P.
Nurse-Midwife
Psychiatric N.C.

B.S. in nursing
RN licensure

6 quarters

University of Minnesota
School of Public Health
1325 Mayo Memorial Building
Minneapolis 55455

Adult N.P.
Family N.S.
Pediatric N.A.

B.S. in nursing
RN licensure
Miller Analogies Test
1 year experience public
  health nursing,
ambulatory child care, or
institutional pediatrics

2 years

MISSOURI

St. Louis University
School of Nursing and Allied
Health Professions
1401 South Grand Boulevard
St. Louis 63104

Cardiovascular N.C.S.
Child N.C.S.
Maternal-Newborn N.C.S.
Medical-Surgical N.C.S.

B.S. in nursing
RN licensure
Miller Analogies Test

3 semesters
1 summer
session

State Address	Area of Concentration (Occupational Title)	Entrance Requirements	Length of Program
University of Missouri School of Nursing Medical Sciences Building Columbia 65201	Clinician	Consult institution	Consult institution
MONTANA Montana State University School of Nursing Bozeman 59715	Cardiac and Respiratory C.S. Chronic Illness and Rehabilitation C.S. Maternal C.S. Medical C.S. Pediatric C.S. Psychiatric C.S. Public Health C.S.	Baccalaureate degree RN licensure GRE	6 quarters
NEBRASKA University of Nebraska Medical Center College of Nursing 42nd and Dewey Omaha 68105	Medical-Surgical C.N.S. Psychiatric C.N.S.	B.S. in nursing RN licensure GRE	3 semesters
NEW JERSEY Rutgers University, The State University of New Jersey Graduate Program University Heights Campus New Brunswick 08903	Psychiatric C.N.S.	B.S. in nursing RN licensure	4 semesters

NEW YORK

State University of New York
at Buffalo
School of Nursing
Health Sciences Building
113 Norton Circle
Buffalo 14214

Adult Health N.C.
Child Health N.C.
Community Health N.C.
Maternal Health N.C.
Psychiatric N.C.
Rehabilitation N.C.

B.S. in nursing
RN licensure

3 semesters

Adelphi University
School of Nursing
Garden City
Long Island 11530

Medical-Surgical C.N.S.
Psychiatric C.N.S.

B.S. in nursing
RN licensure
Plan A—NLN Graduate
Nurse Examination
Miller Analogies Test

2 academic
years

Hunter College of The City
University of New York
School of Nursing
695 Park Avenue
New York 10021

Psychiatric-Mental Health N.C.

B.S. in nursing
RN licensure
GRE

3 semesters

New York University
Division of Nurse Education
Washington Square
New York 10003

Biophysical-Pathology N.C.
Child Psychiatry N.C.
Parent-Child N.C.
Psychiatric-Mental Health N.C.
Public Health N.C.
Rehabilitation N.C.

B.S. in nursing
RN licensure
Plan D—NLN Graduate
Examination

4 semesters

State Address	Area of Concentration (Occupational Title)	Entrance Requirements	Length of Program
Columbia University Graduate Program in Maternity Nursing and Midwifery Department of Nursing Faculty of Medicine Columbia-Presbyterian Medical Center 622 West 168th Street New York 10032	Nurse-Midwife	B.S. in nursing RN licensure 1 year obstetrical nursing experience Miller Analogies Test	12 months
Pace University Graduate School of Nursing 861 Bedford Road Pleasantville 10570	Family N.P.	B.S. in nursing GRE	2 years
University of Rochester School of Medicine and Dentistry Department of Nursing Rochester 14620	Family Health N.C. Medical-Surgical Clinician Psychiatric Clinician	B.S. in nursing RN licensure GRE	3 semesters
Syracuse University School of Nursing 426 Ostrum Avenue Syracuse 13210	Medical-Surgical N.C.	B.S. in nursing RN licensure Miller Analogies Test	4 semesters

NORTH CAROLINA			
University of North Carolina School of Nursing Chapel Hill 27514	Maternal-Child N.C. Medical-Surgical N.C. Obstetrical N.C. Pediatric N.C. Psychiatric N.C. Public Health N.C.	B.S. in nursing RN licensure	4 semesters
University of North Carolina School of Public Health Department of Public Health Nursing Chapel Hill 27514	Public Health N.C.	B.S. in nursing RN licensure GRE	2 semesters 1 summer session
OHIO			
Case Western Reserve University Frances Payne Bolton School of Nursing 2121 Abington Road Cleveland 44106	Maternity N.C. Medical N.C. Pediatric N.C. Psychiatric N.C. Public Health N.C.	B.S. in nursing RN licensure Miller Analogies Test	4 semesters
Ohio State University School of Nursing 1585 Neil Avenue Columbus 43210	Medical-Surgical C.S. Pediatric C.S. Psychiatric-Mental Health C.S.	B.S. in nursing RN licensure	5-6 quarters
University of Cincinnati College of Nursing and Health 3110 Vine Street Cincinnati 45219	Adult Psychiatric N.C. Child Psychiatric N.C. Gerontological N.C. Medical-Surgical N.C.	B.S. in nursing RN licensure Miller Analogies Test Plan A—NLN Graduate Nurse Examination	6 quarters

State Address	Area of Concentration (Occupational Title)	Entrance Requirements	Length of Program
PENNSYLVANIA University of Pennsylvania School of Nursing 205 South 34th Street Philadelphia 19104	Family N.P. Maternity N.C. Medical-Surgical N.C. Pediatric N.C. Psychiatric N.C.	B.S. in nursing RN licensure GRE	4 semesters
University of Pittsburgh School of Nursing Scaife Hall 3550 Terrace Street Pittsburgh 15213	Maternity N.C. Medical-Surgical N.C. Pediatric N.C. Psychiatric-Mental Health N.C.	B.S. in nursing RN licensure Miller Analogies Test	4–5 terms
Pennsylvania State University Department of Nursing 114 Human Development Building University Park 16802	Adult Health N.C. Aging Specialist Community Health N.C. Family Health Specialist Rural Health Specialist	B.S. in nursing RN licensure GRE	5–6 terms
TEXAS Texas Woman's University College of Nursing Box 23026 TWU Station Denton 76204	Community Health N.C. Maternal-Child N.C. Medical-Surgical N.C. Psychiatric-Mental Health N.C.	B.S. in nursing RN licensure	2 semesters and 2 summer sessions

UTAH University of Utah School of Nursing 25 South Medical Drive Salt Lake City 84112	Child Psychiatric C.S. Maternal and Newborn N.C. Medical-Surgical N.C. Nurse-Midwife Psychiatric N.C.S.	B.S. in nursing RN licensure Miller Analogies Test NLN Graduate Nurse Examination	6–7 quarters
VIRGINIA Virginia Commonwealth University School of Nursing Richmond 23219	Maternal N.C. Medical-Surgical N.C. Pediatric N.C. Psychiatric-Mental Health N.C.	B.S. in nursing RN licensure GRE	3 semesters and 1 summer session
WASHINGTON University of Washington School of Nursing Health Sciences Building Seattle 98105	Family and Community N.C. Maternal-Child N.C. Physiological N.C. Psychosocial N.C.	B.S. in nursing RN licensure GRE	4 or 5 quarters
WISCONSIN University of Wisconsin School of Nursing 1402 University Avenue Madison 53706	Medical-Surgical N.C. Pediatric N.C. Psychiatric-Mental Health N.C.	B.S. in nursing RN licensure GRE	3–4 semesters

States With Legislation Sanctioning
Physician's Assistants and Medex

State	Type of law and year enacted	Regulatory agency	Power to make rules	Approval of physician assistant or medex	Job description
Alabama	Regulatory authority, 1971	Board of medical examiners	Yes	Yes	Yes
Alaska	Regulatory authority, 1971	Board of medical examiners	Yes	Yes	—
Arizona	Regulatory authority, 1972	Board of medical examiners, board of osteopathic examiners	Yes	Yes	—
Arkansas	General delegatory, 1971	—	—	—	—
California	Regulatory authority, 1970	Board of medical examiners	Yes	Yes	Yes
Colorado	General delegatory, 1963	—	—	—	—
Connecticut	General delegatory, 1971	—	—	—	—
Delaware	General delegatory, 1971	—	—	—	—
Florida	Regulatory authority, 1971	Board of medical examiners	Yes	Yes	Yes
Georgia	Regulatory authority, 1972	Board of medical examiners	Yes	Yes	Yes
Hawaii	Regulatory authority 1973	Board of medical examiners	Yes	Yes	—
Idaho	Regulatory authority, 1972	Board of medical examiners	Yes	Yes	—
Iowa	Regulatory authority, 1971	Board of medical examiners	Yes	Yes	Yes
Kansas	General delegatory 1964	—	—	—	—
Maine	Regulatory authority 1973	Board of registration in medicine	—	—	—
Maryland	Regulatory authority, 1972	Board of medical examiners	—	—	—

Activities prohibited	Certification renewal	Physician assistant or medex per physician	Education program approved	Approval of physician	Report to legislature
Optometry	—	—	Yes	Yes	—
—	—	—	Yes	—	—
Chiropractics, dentistry, optician's services, naturopathy, optometry, pharmacy	—	—	—	—	—
Optometric services	—	—	—	—	—
Dentistry, dental hygiene, optometry	Annual	2	Yes	Yes	1972
—	—	—	—	—	—
Dentistry, dental hygiene, optometry	—	—	—	—	—
Optometry	—	—	—	—	—
—	Annual	2	Yes	Yes	1973
Pharmacy	—	2	Yes	Yes	—
Optometry	—	—	Yes	—	—
Pharmacy, dentistry, dental hygiene, optometry	—	—	Yes	Yes	—
Optometry	Annual	2	Yes	Yes	1973
—	—	—	—	—	—
Optometry	—	—	—	—	—
—	—	—	—	—	—

State	Type of law and year enacted	Regulatory agency	Power to make rules	Approval of physician assistant or medex	Job description
Massachusetts	Regulatory authority, 1973	Board of approval and certification of physician assistant programs	Yes	—	—
Michigan	Regulatory authority, 1973	Department of health	Yes	—	—
Montana	General delegatory, 1970	—	—	—	—
Nebraska	Regulatory authority, 1973	Board of medical examiners	Yes	Yes	Yes
Nevada	Regulatory authority, 1973	Board of medical examiners	Yes	Yes	—
New Hampshire	Regulatory authority, 1971	Board of medical examiners	Yes	Yes	—
New Mexico	Regulatory authority, 1973	Board of medical examiners	Yes	Yes	—
New York	Regulatory authority 1971	Commissioner of health, commissioner of education	Yes	Yes	—
North Carolina	Regulatory authority, 1971	Board of medical examiners	Yes	Yes	—
Oklahoma	Regulatory authority, 1972	Board of medical examiners	Yes	Yes	—
Oregon	Regulatory authority, 1971	Board of medical examiners	Yes	Yes	Yes
South Carolina	Regulatory authority, 1974	Board of medical examiners	Yes	Yes	—
Tennessee	General delegatory, 1973	—	—	—	—
Utah	Regulatory authority, 1971	Medical association	—	—	—

Activities prohibited	Certification renewal	Physician assistant or medex per physician	Education program approved	Approval of physician	Report to legislature
Chiropractics, dentistry, dental hygiene, optometry, ophthalmology, podiatry	—	2	Yes	—	Annual
—	—	—	Yes	—	Annual
—	—	—	—	—	—
—	Annual	2	Yes	Yes	Annual
Chiropractics, dentistry, optometry, podiatry, hearing aid specialists	—	1	Yes	Yes	—
Optometry, optician's services	—	—	—	—	—
Optometry, podiatry	Annual	2	—	—	—
—	Biennial	2	Yes	—	—
—	Annual	2	Yes	Yes	—
Optometry	—	—	Yes	—	—
Optometry, nursing, dentistry, dental hygiene	Annual	1	Yes	Yes	1973
Optometry	—	—	—	—	—
—	—	—	—	—	—
—	—	—	Yes	Yes	—

State	Type of law and year enacted	Regulatory agency	Power to make rules	Approval of physician assistant or medex	Job description
Vermont	Regulatory authority, 1972	Agency of human services	Yes	Yes	—
Virginia	Regulatory authority, 1973	Board of medical examiners	Yes	Yes	Yes
Washington	Regulatory authority, 1971	Board of medical examiners	Yes	Yes	Yes
West Virginia	Regulatory authority, 1971	Medical licensing board	Yes	Yes	Yes
Wisconsin	Regulatory authority 1973	Board of medical examiners	Yes	Yes	—
Wyoming	Regulatory authority, 1973	Board of medical examiners	Yes	Yes	Yes

*Report to the Congress, from The Comptroller General of the United States, "Progress and Problems in Training and Use of Assistants to Primary Care Physicians," April 8, 1975, pp. 53-55. U.S. General Accounting Office, Washington, D.C.

Note: The table is reproduced from Health Services Reports, Vol. 88, No. 1, January 1973.

Activities prohibited	Certification renewal	Physician assistant or medex per physician	Education program approved	Approval of physician	Report to legislature
—	—	—	—	—	1975
—	Annual	2	Yes	Yes	—
Optometry, dentistry dental hygiene, chiropractic services, chiropody	Annual	1	Yes	Yes	—
Pharmacy, optometry	Annual	—	Yes	Yes	—
Chiropractics, dentistry, dental hygiene, optometry, podiatry	Annual	—	Yes	—	Biennial
Optometry	—	2	Yes	Yes	1975

Index

turnover: and dropouts, 70
Tyler, R. W., 67

University of California at Davis, 157
University of Colorado Pediatric Nurse
  Practitioner Program, 8
University of Rochester, 157

Veterans Administration, 2

Wallis, W. A., 65

Washington, 97; Physicians Assistant Law,
  103; University of and cooption, 12; Uni-
  versity of and Medic, 7
White, Kerr, 161
Wisconsin: compensation, 106
Wise, H. B., 67
World Health Organization, 11

Yett, D. W., 69

About the Authors

Alfred M. Sadler, Jr., is Assistant Vice President at The Robert Wood Johnson Foundation, Princeton, New Jersey.

Dr. Sadler was Director of the Yale Physician's Associate Program from 1970 to 1973. During that time he was an Assistant Professor of Surgery and Public Health at the Yale University School of Medicine and directed the Trauma Program of the Department of Surgery—a multidisciplinary approach to emergency medical care.

He served as the first president of the Association of Physician Assistant Programs, is a member of the advisory committee to the National Board of Medical Examiners in preparing a certifying examination for assistants to the primary care physician and is chairman of the eligibility committee of the National Commission on the Certification of Physicians' Assistants.

During his three years at the National Institutes of Health as a commissioned officer in the U.S. Public Health Service, he was engaged in medical-legal and health policy analysis including the preparation and design of the Uniform Anatomical Gift Act which has been enacted in all states. He served as special assistant to Dr. Roger O. Egeberg (Assistant Secretary for Health) for whom he co-authored a report on the licensure and certification of health personnel.

Dr. Sadler is a graduate of Amherst College and Hahnemann Medical School and did postgraduate training in surgery at the Hospital of the University of Pennsylvania. He is a member of Alpha Omega Alpha.

Blair L. Sadler is Assistant Vice President at The Robert Wood Johnson Foundation, Princeton, New Jersey.

Mr. Sadler was an Assistant Professor of Law at Yale University and Co-Director of the Yale Trauma Program from 1970 to 1973. During that period, he served as Counsel to the Yale Physician's Associate Program.

Formerly a Commission member of the Study of Selected Health Education Programs (SASHEP) and the National Advisory Council on Allied Health Manpower, he currently is a member of the advisory committee to the National Board of Medical Examiners in preparing a certifying examination for assistants to the primary care physician.

During his three years at the National Institutes of Health as a commissioned officer in the U.S. Public Health Service, he was engaged in medical-legal and health policy analysis including the preparation and design of the Uniform Anatomical Gift Act which has been enacted in all states. He served as a special assistant to Dr. Roger O. Egeberg (Assistant Secretary for Health) for whom he co-authored a report on the licensure and certification of health personnel.

Mr. Sadler is a graduate of Amherst College and the University of Pennsylvania Law School, is a member of the Pennsylvania Bar, and served as a Law Clerk for two years with the Superior Court of Pennsylvania.

Ann A. Bliss is Assistant Professor at the Department of Surgery, Yale University School of Medicine; and, Senior Program Consultant at The Robert Wood Johnson Foundation, Princeton, New Jersey.

Formerly Research Associate in the Yale Trauma Program and Lecturer to the Yale Physician's Associate Program, she has also taught psychiatric nursing and sociology in the baccalaureate and master's degree nursing programs at SUNY at Buffalo and Niagara University. In addition to having clinical nursing experience, she is a psychiatric social worker whose clinical practice includes psychotherapy of children and adults.

Since 1973 she has been Managing Editor of *The P.A. Journal—A Journal for New Health Practitioners* and recently joined the Editorial Board of JEN (The Journal of Emergency Nursing).

Mrs. Bliss is a member of the American Nurses' Association, The Academy of Certified Social Workers and The Connecticut Society for Clinical Social Work.

A graduate of the Grace-New Haven School of Nursing, she received her B.S. from the University of Pennsylvania, and M.S.S. from Bryn Mawr College.